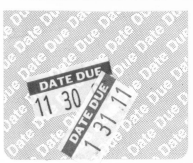

PRENTICE-HALL INTERNATIONAL, INC., *London*
PRENTICE-HALL OF AUSTRALIA, PTY. LTD., *Sydney*
PRENTICE-HALL OF CANADA, LTD., *Toronto*
PRENTICE-HALL OF INDIA PRIVATE LIMITED, *New Delhi*
PRENTICE-HALL OF JAPAN, INC., *Tokyo*

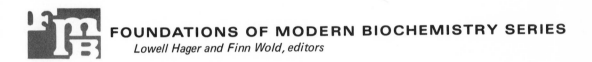

FOUNDATIONS OF MODERN BIOCHEMISTRY SERIES
Lowell Hager and Finn Wold, editors

ORGANIC CHEMISTRY OF BIOLOGICAL COMPOUNDS*
Robert Barker

INTERMEDIARY METABOLISM AND ITS REGULATION
Joseph Larner

PHYSICAL BIOCHEMISTRY
Kensal Edward Van Holde

MACROMOLECULES: STRUCTURE AND FUNCTION
Finn Wold

SPECIAL TOPICS

BIOCHEMICAL ENDOCRINOLOGY OF THE VERTEBRATES
Earl Frieden and Harry Lipner

*Published jointly in Prentice-Hall's *Foundations of Modern Organic Chemistry Series.*

BIOCHEMICAL ENDOCRINOLOGY OF THE VERTEBRATES

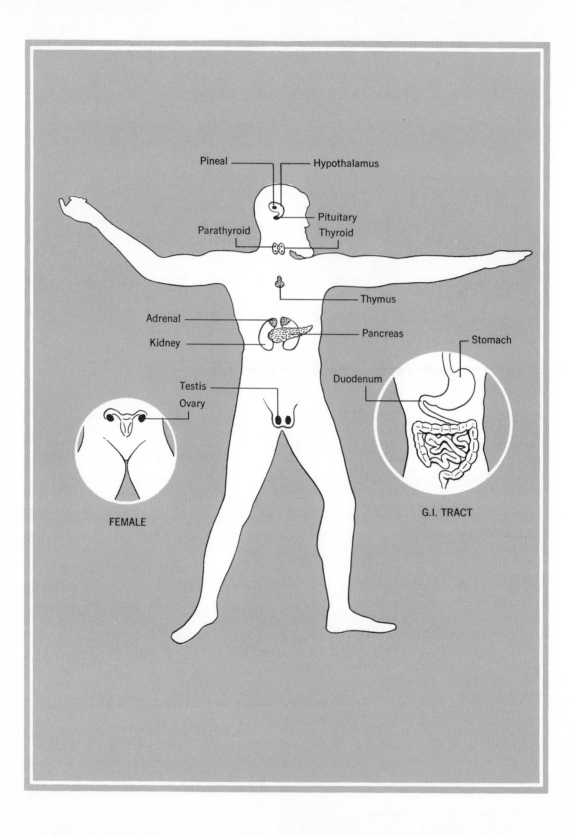

Pineal

Hypothalamus

Pituitary

Parathyroid

Thyroid

Thymus

Adrenal

Pancreas

Kidney

Stomach

Duodenum

Testis

Ovary

FEMALE

G.I. TRACT

BIOCHEMICAL ENDOCRINOLOGY OF THE VERTEBRATES

EARL FRIEDEN

Professor of Chemistry
Florida State University

HARRY LIPNER

Professor of Biology
Florida State University

Prentice-Hall, Inc., Englewood Cliffs, New Jersey

To our patient and understanding wives,
ESTHER and ETHEL

Current printing (last digit)

10 9 8 7 6 5 4 3 2 1

Library of Congress
Catalog Card No. 70-153650

13-076497-3 (C)
13-076489-2 (P)

Printed in the United States of America

PREFACE

As our knowledge of basic biochemistry expands almost explosively, the attention of biological and medical scientists is directed more and more to problems of biochemical control and regulation. Accordingly, the interest in the biochemical messengers, the hormones, which play such a significant role in the regulation of metabolism and development, assumes a greater importance in the field of biochemistry. A compact summary of the basic biochemical facts and ideas concerning endocrinology has long been needed. This has been emphasized by the omission of any significant treatment of the subject of the endocrines in recent textbooks published to cover the field of general biochemistry. We believe that biochemistry curricula should include an appropriate discussion of the endocrines and that this knowledge can best be provided by the availability of an inexpensive, compact, but comprehensive text such as this one.

In recent years, the field of endocrinology and its biochemical implications has grown enormously. Despite the presence of numerous large texts and several series on hormones, there is still need to present the total subject from essentially a biochemical viewpoint. In emphasizing the known biochemical information and ideas of endocrinology and eschewing much speculative material, it is our hope that this text, when supplemented with strategic current references, will remain adequately up to date and useful for a number of years to come.

This book begins with the axioms and generalizations of biochemical endocrinology followed by a discussion of the hypothalamus and the pituitary. Control diagrams are used to clarify and summarize the many complexities of endocrine control and regulation of hormone secretion and target organ response. This is followed by discussion of several hormones having general metabolic effects: thyroid hormones and the pancreatic hormones, insulin and glucagon. The discussion of the effect of the steroid hormones is preceded by a concise analysis of their chemistry, biosynthesis, and structural relationships, treated collectively to emphasize their basic similarities. Then follows a consideration of the action of the steroid hormones: first the more specific sex hormones, then the adrenal steroids, the gluco- and mineral-corticoids, hormones with broad metabolic effects. Included in the latter chapter on the adrenals is a current summary of the biochemistry of the catecholamines originating in the adrenal medulla. The survey of vertebrate hormones is completed by considering those endocrines affecting calcium metabolism and the variety of other hormones found in vertebrates, including the gastrointestinal hormones, melatonin, thymus hormone(s), and the renal hormones. The final chapter is devoted to the correlation and integration of the biochemical effects of these hormones and a general discussion of the various mechanisms of hormone action in the vertebrates.

We are greatly indebted to Drs. Ebert Ashby, Dexter Easton, John Just, and Alan Kent for a critical reading of portions of this manuscript in advance of publication and for valuable suggestions. We also thank Mrs. Molly Beall and Mrs. Lenore Haggard for their cheerful and skillful help in preparing this manuscript.

EARL FRIEDEN
HARRY LIPNER

CONTENTS

ONE | INTRODUCTION TO BIOCHEMICAL ENDOCRINOLOGY

The metazoan in the course of its evolution has developed both neural and hormonal systems to enable it to cope with the complexities of its environment. The neural system contains receptor elements that detect changes in the external or internal environment and transmit information about these changes to effectors which bring about the necessary organismic reactions. The hormonal system is composed of cells that discharge their contents to the internal fluid environment of the organism, thus affecting cell behavior. In developing organisms, hormonal activity is manifested through the regulation of metamorphosis and, at later stages, through the regulation of growth. In adult animals, hormones are responsible for the integrated activity of organ systems and subsystems. They. alter cellular function in response to variation in the external environment, they induce sustained performance by cells, and they change the level of activity of tissues and organs, maintaining constancy of composition within the internal environment. However, since cell activities are stereotyped, neither neural nor hormonal stimuli can induce new activities; they can only stimulate or modulate these cellular functions.

1

I.I   ENDOCRINE CELLS

The concept that certain organs produce materials that may affect the activity or growth of other organs and the behavior of organisms has been implicit in biological literature since Paracelsus in the sixteenth century. In 1849, however, Berthold showed that capons could be restored to masculine appearance and behavior by transplantation of a testis from another rooster. By the end of the nineteenth century, it was clear that a number of organs produced special excitatory substances and released them directly into the circulation. Then Bayliss and Starling (1904) showed that the mucosal lining of the stomach and duodenum contained a substance, extractable with dilute HC1, which could cause the pancreas to secrete pancreatic juice when administered intravenously. They named this substance secretin; for the class of substances which it represented they introduced the name *hormone* (Gr. *hormon:* to rouse, excite). We now know that the sources of hormones are organs of internal secretion called *endocrine glands* (Gr. *endon:* within; *krino:* to separate).

Specific substances attributed to a certain endocrine gland have been traced to particular cells within that gland. For example, the pancreas contains groups of clearly demarcated cells called islets, which produce the pancreatic hormones. These islets consist of two cellular types, called a and β cells, which are the sources of glucagon and insulin, respectively.

Endocrine cells may either store secretions as inactive granules within their cytoplasm (as do the pituitary cells) or as a clear, proteinaceous mass in a cavity surrounded by the secretory cells (as in the case of the thyroid acini). Some secretory cells are derived from neural crest cells, which also produce neural tissue. The cells composing neural tissue possess the ability both to conduct an electrical impulse and to secrete at their termini substances (*neurohumors*) that excite adjacent cells. The secretory cells derived from embryonic neural tissue have lost (or never developed) the ability to conduct an impulse. Examples of such cells are the chromaffin cells which compose the adrenal medulla and produce the catecholamines, norepinephrine, and epinephrine. The most elaborate type of secretory cells, neurosecretory cells, is both conductive and secretory. Their secretions may be classified as *neurohormones* if they enter the body fluids or circulation before encountering their target cells. Examples of neurosecretory cells are found in the hypothalamus of vertebrates.

1.2   CHEMICAL REGULATORS OF CELL FUNCTION

Almost any chemical substance may affect the activities of cells or whole organisms. These substances may be either *exogenous* (originating from without) or *endogenous* (originating from within) in relation to the cells or organisms.

Exogenous substances.

In the external environment of an organism exogenous substances may initiate a broad spectrum of responses through excitation of a small number of receptor cells. They may be introduced into the organism by ingestion or by parenteral administration. Within the organism they become rate-limiting substrates or component parts of cells in the form of enzymes, coenzymes, cofactors, or substances contributing to the maintenance of the ionic composition of the extra- and intracellular environment. The variety of substances that fall within this category is legion; however, they may be grouped as follows:

Nutrient substances include carbohydrates, proteins (and their constituent amino acids), lipids, vitamins, trace elements, and ions (for example, Na^+, K^+, Ca^{2+}, Mg^{2+}).

Pheromones are a group of ill-defined substances that may induce marked behavioral changes. The best-known examples of this group of substances are the sex attractants produced by some female insects (roaches and moths) and the queen substance (9-oxodecenoic acid), which inhibits development of ovaries in worker bees. These substances may serve a communication role, as seen in the case of the evanescent trail substance of fire ants that marks the way to a food source. Newly mated female mice, exposed to a strange male of a different strain, his cage, or his excrement, fail to implant fertilized eggs due to a substance emitted by that male.

Pharmacological substances may act very specifically upon cell structures or enzymes. Examples are the antihistamines, which compete with histamine for receptor sites on cells, or anticholinesterases, which interact with acetylcholine esterase.

Endogenous substances.

These substances may be divided into three categories:

Hormones are systemic-acting substances produced by specialized cells and released into the circulation; they exert relatively specific effects, either on all cells or only on certain cells in specific organs. For example, the effect of testosterone in most somatic cells is to increase protein synthesis, and in seminiferous-tubule epithelium of the testis, to maintain sperm formation.

Tissue factors or *autocoids* are substances generally released in and acting upon highly restricted areas. In this group of substances are histamine, 5-hydroxytryptamine, and the kinins, a group of polypeptides (bradykinin and kallidin). Their release is stimulated by hormones, metabolic products, or cell enzymes.

Intracellular-acting substances may be formed by stimuli acting upon cells to induce the formation of a substance that amplifies the hormone signal and thus increases the activity that characterizes the response of the cell to the hormone. (Such a substance has been called the "second messenger" by Sutherland.) The only known representative of the group is adenosine-cyclic-3′, 5′-monophosphate (c-AMP).

1.3   MECHANISM OF CELL ACTIVATION

The concept of a drug or hormone acting upon a cell to change its level of activity presupposes an interaction of these substances with receptor sites to form complexes. The nature of the receptors and the hormone-receptor complexes are not known; generally the duration of the cellular response is a function of the variable stability of the complex. Such complexes may occur on the cell membrane or inside the cell. Most endocrinologists assume single hormone-receptor interaction for each effect, but since several of the hormones appear to have more than one effect, they may interact with more than one receptor. The hormone-receptor complex may bring about (1) an increase in membrane permeability to allow substrates to enter the cells, (2) the initiation of the formation of a second messenger, or (3) the synthesis of proteins to increase the activity level of one or more enzyme systems (see Chapter 10).

Most cells can function independently of any exogenous controls. There is ample literature indicating that cells have elaborated a series of negative feedback systems in the metabolism of food substances that function effectively without external regulation or influence. The metabolism of carbohydrates, fats, and proteins can take place without glucocorticoids, insulin, glucagon, and growth hormone; however, these substances are necessary to maintain metabolic rates commensurate with the needs of the organism. Furthermore, growth and differentiation beyond the earliest developmental stages are dependent on hormones: growth of most mammals is retarded and metamorphosis of amphibian larval stages does not occur in the absence of thyroid hormones.

1.4   COMPARISON OF HORMONES AND TRACE DIETARY SUBSTANCES

Trace substances derived from the diet and essential to cellular metabolic processes must be distinguished from hormones that exert controls on cellular metabolic processes. Both groups of substances occur in trace amounts in the blood. The blood concentrations of vitamins are generally a function of the quantity of vitamins in the diet, while most hormonal blood concentrations are independent of trace components in food (with the exception of thyroid hormones, which need dietary iodine for their biosynthesis). Many nutrients affect the rate of synthesis and secretion of hormones; for example, blood glucose concentration affects insulin and growth hormone secretion, and protein deprivation affects the synthesis of protein hormones. Vitamins and trace elements are essential to the survival of cells since as cofactors they are essential components of enzymes and structural proteins. In higher vertebrates, certain hormones (insulin, aldosterone, vasopressin, parathyroid hormone) are essential to life; this need has not been established in inframammalian vertebrates. However, hormones do contribute to the optimal functioning of many cells and the overall well-being of these organisms.

Diseases due to hormonal excess or deficiency were identified in antiquity, as were some of the vitamin and trace-element diseases. Dysfunction due to vitamin excess is a relatively rare, modern phenomenon; vitamins A and D have been implicated in several hypervitaminosis diseases. Excess of tissue copper is associated with an inheritable disease, hepatolenticular degeneration (Wilson's disease) and excess of zinc simulates a copper-deficiency disease. The effects of most hormonal excesses have been observed; for example, gigantism and acromegaly are the results of an excess of growth hormone, the former occurring in the growing organism and the latter in the adult. Hormone-deficiency diseases are well-known clinical entities. Examples of these are Addison's disease, due to adrenocortical deficiency, and Gull's disease, caused by deficiency of thyroid hormone.

1.5 PHYSIOLOGICAL PROPERTIES OF HORMONES

Hormones have a number of distinctive properties: (1) They are produced in small amounts by endocrine glands. The amounts secreted range from nanograms to milligrams per day. Their blood concentrations are low and their tissue concentrations are even lower. In mammals, the concentration of thyroxine in plasma is $5 \times 10^{-8} M (4 \mu g/100$ ml) whereas in tadpole tissue it is about 10^{-8} to $10^{-9} M$ (1 to 10 ng/g). (2) In the normal animal, the secretion rate of a hormone is determined by the need for that hormone. The control mechanism is frequently complex and relatively specific for each endocrine gland. (3) Hormones have no direct effect on the organs secreting them; for example, the metabolic and secretory activities of the thyroid gland are apparently unaffected by the thyroid hormone. (4) Hormones may exert effects on cells throughout the organism or they may act on specific target cells in certain organs. Insulin exemplifies the first effect and luteinizing hormone, which acts on the interstitial cell in the gonads of both sexes, illustrates the second. (5) The effect of hormones on tissues is determined largely by the capacity of the tissue to respond and the amount of hormone present. Growth hormone in the young organism induces growth, whereas in the adult it controls the release of free fatty acids from storage sites. If the adult is given an excess of growth hormone, the viscera increases in size and the bones thicken. (6) Hormones act as trigger substances, initiating biochemical reactions that persist after the hormones are no longer detectable. The excess blood sugar (*hyperglycemia*) caused by epinephrine reaches a peak long after the hormone is undetectable in the blood. (7) Although hormones have specific effects in cells, many may have a number of effects. Insulin alters cellular permeability to glucose in many tissues (brain tissue is an exception), but it also increases biosynthesis of proteins in muscle and perhaps other tissues.

1.6 FUNCTION OF HORMONES

Hormones act at the cellular level; the physiological effect of this action is the summated response of a large number of cells constituting an organ. The activity of the organ may alter composition of body fluids, gaseous exchange, or behavior of the cardiovascular or central nervous system.

Regulatory or homeostatic function.

It is a biological truism that one may predict the composition of the body fluids of healthy organisms with an amazing degree of precision and consistency. The concept of an internal fluid environment was formulated by Claude Bernard, the great nineteenth-century French physiologist, and the concept of its precise regulation, *homeostasis,* was proposed by Walter Cannon in the 1920s.

The mechanism by which homeostasis is attained and maintained is now best explained in terms of control theory. The self-adaptive negative-feedback loop is the simplest scheme that allows understanding of the type of regulation involved. One may conceive of a number of such loops acting to insure the constancy of blood-glucose concentrations. Figure 1.1 shows examples of a number of simple negative-feedback loops acting together to cause homeostasis of blood glucose. The glucose concentration in the blood stimulates the pancreas to initiate secretion of either insulin or glucagon. Activation of pancreatic β cells by a high blood sugar level results in secretion of insulin, which facilitates the movement of glucose out of the blood into cells, and also increases the activity of the gluconeogenetic system. Activation of the pancreatic α cells by a low blood sugar concentration causes secretion of glucagon which, by inducing the formation of c-AMP, primarily affects the phosphorylase system of the liver and causes secretion of glucose into the blood. (See Chapter 7.)

Figure 1.1   *(opposite page)* Regulations of blood glucose. Three different pathways are illustrated: (1) Insulin is involved in lowering the blood sugar concentration by inducing a hypoglycemia. (2) Glucagon can raise the blood sugar concentration by inducing a hyperglycemia. The balance between insulin and glucagon results in normal blood sugar levels. (3) Catecholamines (epinephrine and norepinephrine) cause a hyperglycemia, increasing the amounts of substrate so that muscles may show a sustained response to stress. Secretion of catecholamines is caused by increased neural activation of the hypothalamus.

Integrated regulation, via the endocrine system, of the various functions of the organism is most easily illustrated by use of qualitative feedback control diagrams. In all the diagrams of this type, it is assumed that hormone stimulation causes a response that is linear when plotted against the log of the dose of hormone. The curves generally suggest secretory rates. Although the magnitudes of the curves are hypothetical, their directions are based on our interpretation of the literature. For example, the action of glucose on the pancreatic β cell is stimulatory and is illustrated by a curve with a positive slope; the action of glucose on the α cell is assumed to be inhibitory, depressing secretion, and is shown with a negative slope.

Symbols: blood glucose   ↑   = hyperglycemia
blood glucose   ↓   = hypoglycemia
→ → =   controlling system
← ← =   controlled system

(Modified from H. T. Milhorn, Jr., *The Application of Control Theory to Physiological Systems,* W. A. Saunders Co., Philadelphia, 1966.)

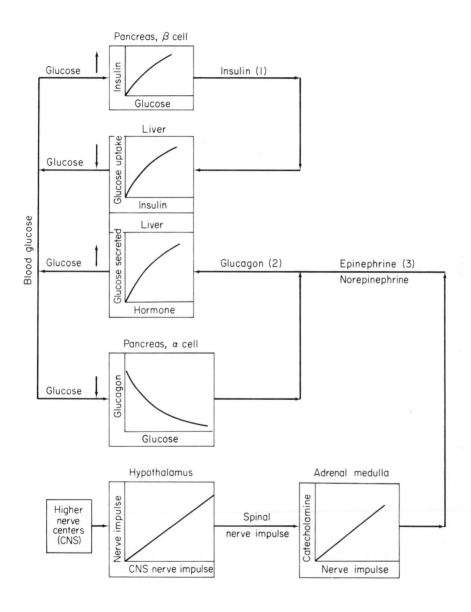

Integrative function.

Hormones provide animals with an integrative capacity that may parallel or supplement the role of the nervous system, as seen in Figure 1.1. Under the stress of fear or anger, the nervous system may activate the hypothalamus and sequentially, by neural impulses, the adrenal medulla. The resulting secretion of catecholamines causes a hyperglycemia by a mechanism similar to that involving glucagon.

Morphogenetic function.

The developing organism requires hormones in its transitions from one stage to another. Larval insects need decreasing amounts of juvenile hormone in each successive developmental stage. Amphibian tadpoles need thyroid hormones to initiate and complete metamorphosis, and young vertebrates need growth hormone for growth and development.

Permissive function.

Cells may be partially or totally unable to respond to the stimulus of a hormone if a second hormone is absent. In the absence of thyroxine, growth hormone is less effective. Epinephrine is unable to elicit an increase in oxygen consumption or blood glucose concentration unless the thyroid gland is functional or thyroxine is administered.

1.7   ENDOCRINE INTEGRATION VERSUS NEURAL INTEGRATION

The function of the endocrine system parallels that of the nervous system, providing for homeostasis, integration, differentiation, and growth. It is therefore interesting to note (Table 1.1) that the organization of the endocrine and nervous systems may be broadly compared. One can describe three levels of complexity in the nervous system involving increasing numbers of neurons. At the simplest level is the *monosynaptic reflex;* an afferent neuron conducts a signal initiated by a stimulus into the spinal cord, where it communicates via a *synapse** with a motor cell (the efferent neuron), which sends its fiber (axon) to the effector cell. An analogous situation is seen in the endocrine system when parathyroid gland cells are stimulated to release parathyroid hormone by a reduction of Ca^{2+} in the circulating blood. The effector cells lowering the Ca^{2+} concentration are osteoclasts of bone and distal convoluted tubule cells of the nephron.

At the second level of complexity in the nervous system is the pathway that includes an interneuron between the afferent and efferent neurons. The interven-

---

*A synapse is the point of contact between contiguous nerve cells generally consisting of nerve endings lying on the cell body. The cell surfaces are separated by 100 to 200 Å. Excitation of the nerve generally results in the release of a neurohumor by the nerve endings and resulting excitation of the contiguous nerve.

TABLE 1.1 COMPARISON BETWEEN NERVOUS SYSTEM AND ENDOCRINE SYSTEM

Generic Designation	Components	Stimulus	Central Organization	Efferent Limb	Efferent Structures
Monosynaptic pathway	Afferent-efferent neuron pathway	Muscle stretch	Spinal cord →	Motor cell →	Muscles
Monohormonal pathway	Single gland system	Change in blood composition (Glucose, Ca²⁺)	Single gland →	Hormones →	Responding tissues
			α- and β- cells of islets of Langerhans Light cell of thyroid and parathyroid glands	Glucagon and insulin Thyrocalcitonin and parathyroid hormone	Liver and muscles Bones and kidney
		NaCl	Supraoptic nucleus of hypothalamus	Vasopressin (antidiuretic hormone)	Kidney
Disynaptic pathway	Afferent neuron-interneuron-efferent neuron pathway	Pain	ο——— Spinal cord ———	——— Motor cell ——→	Muscles
Dihormonal pathway	Two gland system	Inhibition of tonic secretion	Hypothalamus ——→ Pituitary GRH[a] PIH[a] MIH[a]	Hormones ——→ Growth hormone Prolactin Melanocyte stimulating hormone	Responding tissues Body cells Melanocytes
Polysynaptic pathway	Afferent neuron-several interneurons (in sequence)-efferent neuron pathway	Most sensory inputs	ο——→ Spinal Cord ο——→	——— Motor cell ——→	Muscles
Polyhormonal pathway	Several glands in sequence	External factors (light, temperature changes in blood concentration of stimulating compounds)	Secretory cell ——→ Secretory cell ——→ Secretory cell Hypothalamus · Pituitary · Target gland TRH[a] · TSH · Thyroid gland LRH[a] · LH · Corpus luteum FRH[a] · FSH · Ovarian follicle · ACTH · Adrenal cortex	Hormones ——→ Thyroid hormones Progesterone } Estrogen Cortisol	Responding tissues Body cells Uterus and mammary gland Body cells

[a] Abbreviations:
GRH, growth-hormone-releasing hormone;
PIH, prolactin-release-inhibiting hormone;
MIH, melanocyte-stimulating-hormone-inhibiting hormone;

TRH, thyroid-stimulating-hormone-releasing hormone;
LRH, luteinizing-hormone-releasing hormone (interstitial-cell-stimulating hormone);
FRH, follicle-stimulating-hormone-releasing hormone;
CRH, adrenocorticotrophin-releasing hormone.

tion of the interneuron creates a *disynaptic reflex*. In an endocrine pathway the "center" corresponding to the interneuron may be loosely said to consist of all glands that interact regardless of their distances from each other. Analogous to the disynaptic reflex is the action of stimuli on the hypothalamus to regulate secretion of neurohormones that may in turn regulate the adenohypophyseal release of hormones to act on effector cells. For example, hypoglycemia or suckling stimulate the hypothalamus to secrete growth hormone-releasing hormone (GRH) or reduce secretion of prolactin-release-inhibiting hormone (PIH); these hormones affect the secretion of growth hormone (GH) or prolactin by the pituitary.

On the third level of complexity, many interneurons are introduced between the afferent neuron and the effector cell; similarly in the endocrine system, several glands and their secretions may be introduced between the initial stimulus and the response in the effector cell. An example of such a complex system is seen when an animal is subjected to a stress (say, cold, epinephrine, or histamine). The neural activity of the hypothalamus causes the release of corticotrophin-releasing hormone (CRH), stimulating pituitary secretion of adrenocorticotrophic hormone (ACTH); this acts on the adrenal cortex to cause secretion of glucocorticoids as a final response. It should be noted that in this analogy we follow our earlier principle: no matter how dispersed they may be, the component secretory structures constitute a center whose sequential activity provides the essential connection between the stimulus and the response.

It is necessary to note that contrasts as well as parallels exist between the nervous and endocrine systems. Two readily apparent differences are speed of control and degree of autonomy. The nervous system requires only milliseconds from the stimulus to the response, while the endocrine system requires seconds to elicit a response when it is rapid—and more usually, hours or days. The somatic nervous system is largely under conscious control; even the behavior of the autonomic nervous system can be regulated to some extent. The endocrine system, however, is largely independent of conscious regulation.

1.8   CHEMICAL CHARACTERISTICS OF HORMONES

Hormones are derived from three classes of chemical substances: (1) The smallest group is derived from two amino acids: tryptophan, which is converted to serotonin and melatonin; and tyrosine, which is the source of the catecholamines and the thyroid hormones. (2) A larger group of hormones stems from cholesterol and is converted to adrenocortical and gonadal steroids. (3) The largest group of hormones is peptides or proteins. They vary in length from 8 to more than 180 amino acids and may have carbohydrate groups attached to them. Similar hormones from different species administered heterologously induce antibodies. The antigenicity of the protein hormones is due to dissimilarity of amino acid sequences at parts of the molecule not related to the action of the hormone (see discussion of the cortico-trophins). Table 1.2 lists the hormones according to chemical identity, organ of origin, target cell or tissues, and primary functions.

TABLE 1.2 THE VERTEBRATE HORMONES; CLASSES, TARGETS, AND EFFECTS

Hormone	Target	Effects
I. Peptides, Protein Hormones		
1. Pituitary Gland (Hypophysis)		
A. Adenohypophysis		
a. Pars distalis		
growth hormone (GH, somatotrophin)	All tissues	Growth of tissues (easily seen in long bones, metabolism of protein, mobilization of fat)
Adrenocorticotrophin (ACTH, corticotrophin)	Adrenal cortex	Synthesis and release of gluco-corticoids
Thyroid-stimulating hormone (TSH, thyrotrophin)	Adipose tissue Thyroid gland	Lipolysis Synthesis and secretion of thyroxine and triiodothyronine
Male Follicle-stimulating hormone (FSH)	Seminiferous tubules	Production of sperm
Interstitial-cell-stimulating hormones (ICSH, luteinizing hormone, LH)	Testes	Synthesis and secretion of androgens
Female FSH	Ovary (follicles)	Follicle maturation
LH	Ovary (interstitial cells)	Final maturation of follicle, estrogen secretion, ovulation, Corpus luteum formation, Progesterone secretion
Prolactin	Mammary glands (alveolar cell) Crop gland of pigeons	Milk production in prepared gland Crop gland "milk" production
b. Pars intermedia Melanocyte-stimulating hormones (α- and β-MSH, Intermedin)	Melanophores	Pigment dispersal in melanophores (darkening of skin)
B. Neurohypophysis (Posterior lobe)		
Oxytocin (Let-down factor, milk-ejection factor)	Uterus Mammary glands	Contraction of smooth muscle, milk ejection
Vasopressin (antidiuretic hormone, ADH)	Kidney Arteries	Reabsorption of water Contraction of smooth muscle

TABLE 1.2 THE VERTEBRATE HORMONES; CLASSES, TARGETS, AND EFFECTS   (cont.)

Hormone	Target	Effects
2. Pancreas		
Insulin	All cells	Carbohydrate, fat and protein metabolism, hypoglycemia
Glucagon	Liver	Hyperglycemia
3. Ovary		
Relaxin	Pelvic ligaments	Separation of pelvic bones
4. Thyroid		
Thyrocalcitonin (calcitonin)	Bones, kidney	Excretion of calcium and phosphorus, inhibited calcium release from bones, decreased blood calcium levels
5. Parathyroid		
Parathyroid hormone	Bones, kidney	Elevated blood calcium and phosphorus levels, mobilization of calcium from bone, inhibited calcium excretion from kidney
6. Kidney[a]		
Erythropoietin	Bone marrow	Increased erythrocyte production
Renin	Adrenal cortex	Aldosterone-synthesis, secretion
7. Stomach and Duodenum		
Gastrin	Stomach	Acid secretion
Enterogastrone	Stomach	Inhibited gastric mobility
Cholecystokinin	Gall bladder	Contraction of the gall bladder
Secretin	Pancreas	Secretion of water and salts
Pancreozymin	Pancreas	Secretion of digestive enzymes
II. Amino Acid Derivatives		
1. Thyroid		
Thyroxin Triiodothyronine	Most cells	Increased metabolic rate, growth, and development
2. Adrenal Medulla		
Norepinephrine Epinephrine	Most cells	Increased cardiac activity, Elevated blood pressure, Glycolysis, hyperglycemia
3. Pineal gland		
Melatonin	Melanophores	Dispersion of melanin

[a]The renal hormones appear to be enzymes that activate plasma subtrates, which act on the target organ.

TABLE 1.2 THE VERTEBRATE HORMONES; CLASSES, TARGETS, AND EFFECTS   (cont.)

Hormone	Target	Effects

4. Argentaffin cells, platelets, nerves
    Serotonin
    (5-hydroxy-tryptamine)
	Arterioles, central nervous system	Vasoconstriction

III. Steroids and Lipids
  1. Testes
      Androgen (testosterone)
	Most cells	Development and maintenance of masculine characteristics and behavior

2. Ovary Estrogen (estradiol−17β)	Most cells	Development and maintenance of feminine characteristics and behavior
3. Corpus luteum Progesterone	Uterus, mammary glands	Maintenance of uterine endometrium and stimulation of mammary duct formation

4. Adrenal cortex
      Hydrocortisone
      Cortisone
	Most cells	Balanced carbohydrate, protein, and fat metabolism; anti-inflammatory action

Aldosterone	Kidney	Reabsorption of Na^+ from urine

5. Prostate, Seminal Vesicles,
  Brain, Nerves
      Prostaglandins
	Uterus, rabbit duodenum	Contraction of smooth muscle

1.9 THE EXPERIMENTAL APPROACH TO ENDOCRINOLOGY

The discipline known as endocrinology initially evolved from the establishment of the relationship of pathology in certain organs to particular disease states. In 1855 Addison recognized a relationship between low blood pressure, muscular weakness, weight loss, bronzing of skin, and pathology of the adrenal gland. In 1879 Gull related dry skin, sparse hair, puffiness of the face and hands, and swollen tongue to myxedema, the pathological deficiency of thyroid function in adults; in 1871 Hilton-Fagge related the cretinoid state to a congenital inadequacy of thyroid function in early childhood.

A system of general experimental techniques evolved concurrent to these clinical studies. The laboratory analysis of hormone action has led to a recognition of pathological states not known before and to a better understanding of the endocrine system and its pathological physiology. Endocrinology has also brought about rational treatment of dysfunctions of endocrine glands and a broader understanding of the general biochemistry and physiology of living systems.

The laboratory study of endocrinology required that many of the pathological conditions observed in man be duplicated in experimental animals. Certain of these conditions have been induced experimentally by surgical removal of specific organs, indicating the relationship of the organ involved to the pathological state. The first experiment of this kind, demonstrating the role of the testis in masculine behavior, was conducted by Berthold.

Historically, there is a parallelism in the acquisition of knowledge about each of the vertebrate hormones that extends from the recognition and description of the pathological state to the discovery of the hormone. Such observations have been followed by the development of assay techniques, the isolation of active ingredients, and their subsequent purification, identification, and synthesis. Efforts to explain their mechanisms of action have been made with indifferent results until recently. More productive have been those studies which have elucidated the integrated mechanisms that maintain the internal environment during metabolism. Table 1.3 indicates the usual steps in studying an endocrine gland and its secretion.

TABLE 1.3 STEPS IN THE STUDY OF HORMONES AND THEIR ACTIONS

1. Demonstration that an organ has an endocrine role in the economy of the organism:
   a. Create a deficit by surgical or chemical removal of the organ
   b. Relieve the deficit by administering crude extracts or by transplanting organ
   c. Induce hyperactive states by giving extracts for a long time, with large amounts of material, or by transplanting several of the organs into a single recipient

2. Determination of the chemical nature of the active material:
   a. Conduct bioassay or equivalent chemical tests for hormonal activity
   b. Isolate and purify
   c. Identify and synthesize

3. Determination of the mechanism of biosynthesis and secretion of hormone:
   a. Analyze the biosynthetic pathway
   b. Control secretion by chemical means

4. Determination of the mechanism of hormone action:
   a. Determine the number and kind of effects
   b. Determine the target tissue
   c. Determine the target site in the affected cell
   d. Analyze the effect at the molecular level

REFERENCES

Gorbman, A., and H. A. Bern: *A Textbook of Comparative Endocrinology,* John Wiley & Sons, New York, 1962.

Harris, R. S., I. G. Wool, and J. A. Loraine (eds.): *Vitamins and Hormones,* 1–26, Academic Press, New York, 1943–1968.

Recent Progr. Hormone Res., 1–26, Academic Press, New York, 1945–1970.

TWO | HORMONES OF THE PITUITARY AND HYPOTHALAMUS

2.1 THE PITUITARY GLAND AND THE HYPOTHALAMUS

The pituitary gland, or *hypophysis cerebri*, is an unpaired organ located on the floor of the skull and connected to the brain by a stalk. It is one of the most important of the glands in the organism; by secretion of ten hormones, it directly regulates the activity of many endocrine glands and indirectly regulates the others. The naming of its three anatomical areas and their subdivisions has become somewhat complex and is illustrated in Figure 2.1. An evagination from the roof of the primitive oral cavity (Rathke's pouch) contributes the epithelial cells that will eventually become the adenohypophysis. A similar outgrowth (the infundibulum) from what will be the floor of the third ventricle contributes the neural elements that will constitute the neurohypophysis. The pars tuberalis and pars distalis are the source of seven anterior lobe hormones. The pars intermedia, which produces another hormone (melanophore-stimulating hormone), appears in some species as a clearly delineated area separated from the pars distalis by a narrow cleft, the remnant of Rathke's pouch.

The secretory cells of the adenohypophysis are extensively supplied with capil-

15

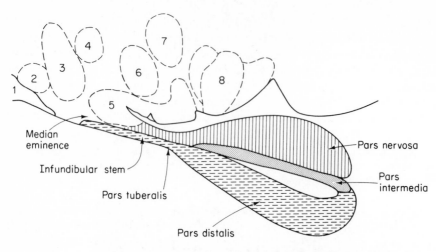

Median eminence

Infundibular stem

Pars tuberalis

Pars distalis

Pars nervosa

Pars intermedia

Figure 2.1 Highly schematized diagram of the hypophysis and some areas of the hypothalamus. Particular note should be taken of the median eminence, the area
through which the hypothalamo-hypophyseal tract passes on its way from
the hypothalamic nuclei to the neurohypophysis; axons of other nuclei
terminate in the median eminence on the capillaries of the hypothalamo-
hypophyseal portal system. Areas of the hypothalamus are noted as follows: (1) optic chiasma; (2) supra chiasma; (3) anterior hypothalamic area;
(4) paraventricular nucleus; (5) arcuate nucleus; (6) ventromedial nucleus;
(7) dorsomedial nucleus; (8) medial mammillary nucleus. The relationship
of the areas of the hypophysis to each other are listed below.

Major anatomical areas	Anatomical subdivisions	Functional areas
Anterior lobe	Pars distalis Pars tuberalis	Adenohypophysis
Posterior lobe	Pars intermedia Pars nervosa	
Hypophyseal stalk	Infundibular stem Median eminence	Neurohypophysis

laries. The neurohypophysis contains nerve fibers and pituicytes (one of several
types of nonneural central nervous system connective tissue cells collectively called
neuroglia). The nerve fibers project from the hypothalamus into the neurohypophysis, where they comprise the hypothalamo-hypophyseal tract, and terminate
on capillaries. Neurosecretory granules are formed in the cell bodies composing the
hypothalamic nuclei (supraoptic and paraventricular) and are transported through
the nerve fibers into the neurohypophysis, where they are stored in the nerve
terminals which rest on the capillaries. The following discussion deals with the
synthesis, secretion, and action of the ten pituitary hormones.

Adenohypophyseal Cytology

The adenohypophysis contains at least six different cell types, each with its own
secretion. These cells may be differentiated by staining and fluorescent antibody

techniques, as well as by size and composition of their granules, localization in the gland, and cyclical activity; they are also characterized by their relationship to pregnancy, lactation, and the pathological states caused by thyroidectomy, castration, adrenalectomy, gigantism, and dwarfism. Lipoptrophin (β and γ) is the only adenohypophyseal hormone to which a cell type is not assigned. Table 2.1 lists the adenohypophyseal hormones according to general class of secretory cells, specific cell types, and average granule diameters, as seen in mammals and most vertebrates.

Anatomical Organization of the Regulatory System of Adenohypophyseal Secretion

Secretory activity of adenohypophyseal cells is regulated by hormones produced in the hypothalamus and delivered to the cells through a specialized vascular pathway. There is no neural pathway between the hypothalamus and the adenohypophysis. Until recently the mechanism for regulation of pituitary secretion was assumed to be a negative-feedback system between the pituitary and the gland under its control. This idea evolved into the concept of the thyroid-pituitary, adrenal-pituitary, and gonad-pituitary axes. These relationships dominated the field of endocrine regulation until the anatomical distribution of blood vessels between the pituitary and hypothalamus was recognized in 1930 and the direction of the blood flow in this vascular system was established in 1936. Two sets of capillaries were observed, connected by vessels which passed over the surface of the pituitary stalk. One capillary bed was described in the median eminence and the other in the adenohypophysis (Figure 2.2). Blood flowing from an arterial source into the bed in the median eminence was collected by portal vessels and distributed to another bed around the secretory cells of the adenohypophysis. The significance of this observation was unappreciated until Harris's brilliant demonstration in 1948 that

TABLE 2.1 ADENOHYPOPHYSEAL HORMONES, CELL TYPE, AND GRANULE SIZES[a]

	Cell Type		Size of Granules, $m\mu$
Hormone	*General*	*Specific*	
Growth hormone (GH somototrophin)	Acidophil[b]	Somatotroph	350
Prolactin (luteotrophin)	Acidophil	Mammotroph	600
Thyroid-stimulating hormone (TSH)	Basophil	Thyrotroph	140
Follicle-stimulating hormone (FSH)	Basophil	Gonadotroph	200
Luteinizing hormone (LH)	Basophil	Gonadotroph	200
Adrenocorticotrophic hormone (ACTH)	Chromophobe	Corticotroph	200

[a] Modified from W. C. Hymer and W. H. McShan, *J. Cell Biol.,* **17**, 67 (1963).

[b] Ehrlich divided stains into those with affinities for nuclear constituents and for cytoplasmic constituents. Later workers showed that basic (cationic) dyes (for example, methylene blue, azure A and B) stain structures composed of nucleic acids, sulfated polysaccharides, sialic and uronic polysaccharides, or negatively charged proteins, whereas the acidic (anionic) dyes (for example, eosin Y and B, orange Y) react with positively charged proteins. The terms *basophil, acidophil,* and *chromophobe* were assigned respectively to the cells with cytoplasmic granules that stain with basic dyes, acidic dyes, and neutral dye.

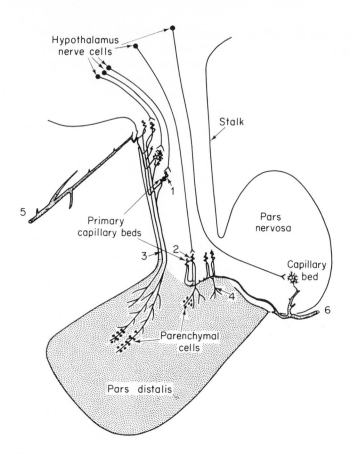

Hypothalamus
nerve cells

Stalk

5

1

Primary
capillary beds

Pars
nervosa

3   2

Capillary
bed

4

6

Parenchymal
cells

Pars distalis

Figure 2.2   Diagram showing some of the possible neurovascular connections between
hypothalamic nuclei and the pituitary gland. Pathways are shown between
nerve cells in the hypothalamus and parenchymal cells around sinusoids in
the pars distalis. The axons of these nerve cells terminate on convoluted
vessels of the primary capillary bed in the neural tissue of the stalk (1) or
in the lower infundibular stem (2). Here the postulated neurohormones are
believed to be transferred into the blood stream, and are then carried to
specific groups of anterior lobe cells by the long (3) or short (4) portal
vessels. Another pathway is shown between a hypothalamic nerve cell and
the capillary bed of the pars nervosa. (5), superior hypophyseal artery; (6),
inferior hypophyseal artery. [From J. H. Adams, P. M. Daniel, and M. M.
L. Prichard, "Distribution of Hypophyseal Portal Blood in the Anterior
Lobe of the Pituitary Gland," *Endocrinol*, **75**, 120 (1964).]

the portal vessels must be intact for regulation of pituitary secretion; for example,
the rabbit, which normally ovulates 10 hr after mating, did not ovulate when the
pituitary stalk was severed and interposing materials (waxed paper, or aluminum
foil) prevented regeneration of the vessels. Long and short portal vessels are shown
in Figure 2.2, each with its specific area of origin (in the median eminence or
pituitary stalk) and termination (in the adenohypophysis). Since the various types
of secretory cells in the adenohypophysis have relatively discrete locations it is
probable that a highly specific, point-to-point neurovascular relationship exists.

However, an even greater and more specific hypothalamic control was demonstrated by the discovery of hypothalamic releasing hormones, which regulate synthesis and secretion of each secretory cell type in the adenohypophysis.

Neurohormonal Regulation of Secretory Activity

Regulation of adenohypophyseal cells is achieved by blood-borne substances introduced into the capillaries of the hypothalamo-hypophyseal portal system at the median eminence. At present, each cell in the adenohypophysis is thought to be under the influence of at least one regulator substance. Seven such substances—five activators and two inhibitors—have now been described (Table 2.2). They are

TABLE 2.2 SOME MAMMALIAN HYPOTHALAMIC NEUROHORMONES[a]

Hypothalamic Hormone	New Abbreviation	Old Abbreviation	Chemical Nature	Minimal Active Dose[b] (dry weight)	
				In Vivo	In Vitro
Corticotrophin-releasing hormone	CRH	CRF	Polypeptide?	1 μg	a few ng[c]
Luteinizing hormone-releasing hormone	LRH or LH-RH	LRF or LH-RF	Not a polypeptide?	1 ng	a few ng
Follicle-stimulating hormone-releasing hormone	FRH or FSH-RH	FSH-RF	Polyamine derivative?	4 ng	a few ng
Thyroid-stimulating-hormone-releasing-hormone[d]	TRH	TRF	Not a simple polypeptide?	1 ng	0.01 ng
Growth-hormone-releasing hormone or somatotrophin-releasing hormone	GRH or SRH	GRF or SRF	Probably polypeptide	12 ng	a few ng
Prolactin-release-inhibiting-hormone	PIH or PRIH	PIF	Unknown	< 1 mg	< 1 mg
MSH-release-inhibiting hormone	MIH or MRIH	MIF	Not a polypeptide	60 ng	6 ng

[a] Adapted from A. V. Schally, W. Locke, A. J. Kastin, and C. Y. Bowers, "Some aspects of Neuroendocrinology," in T. B. Schwartz (ed.), *Year Book of Endocrinology,* Year Book Medical Publishers, Chicago, 1968, pp. 5-29. Used by permission of Year Book Medical Publishers.

[b] As of March, 1968.

[c] 1 ng = 1 millimicrogram.

[d] Pyroglutamyl-histidyl-proline:

growth-hormone-releasing hormone (GRH), corticotrophin-releasing hormone (CRH), thyroid-stimulating-hormone-releasing hormone (TRH), follicle-stimulating-hormone-releasing hormone (FRH), luteinizing-hormone-releasing hormone (LRH), prolactin-release-inhibiting hormone (PIH), and melanocyte-stimulating-hormone-release-inhibiting hormone (MIH). There are indications that other inhibitory factors may exist.

As yet, relatively little is known about the group of hypothalamic substances collectively called releasing hormones. Tissue extractions have shown them to be in the hypothalamus but not in the other areas of the brain. Although they have been studied intensively, the structure of only one has been determined. Fractionations and column separations suggest that some releasing factors are polypeptides, whereas others are unidentified or described as polyamine derivatives. Most of the recent information about them is summarized in Table 2.2. Hypothalamic releasing hormones have been classified as *neurohormones* rather than *neurohumors,* since unlike the latter, which are released at nerve endings and activate adjacent nerve bodies, they are released into the blood and activate cells some distance from their point of release. The neurosecretory cells are reported to have at their terminals two different sized granules, large ones composed of neurosecretory substances and small ones containing neurohumoral substances. It has been proposed that nerve impulses activate the release of the neurohumor, facilitating the discharge of neurohormone.

The cells that produce releasing hormones serve as an intermediate structure between the nervous system and the endocrine system (see Figure 2.3). They may be considered as *transducer cells*, transforming neural to hormonal signals. As yet unanswered is the question of whether the cell is merely a transducer, receiving the signal from a receptor cell, or whether it is both receptor and transducer. The significance of the neurosecretory mechanism (Figure 2.3) is that it allows environmental stimuli perceived in the central nervous system to exert effects on the endocrine system. Furthermore, it acts as a vigilant controlling system integrating many of the secretory and metabolic processes of the organism.

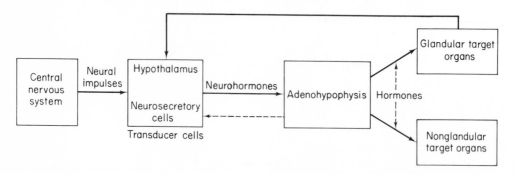

Figure 2.3   The neurosecretory regulation of hormone secretion. The relationship between the periphery and the central nervous system is schematized to emphasize that these operate under feedback control regulation. Short loops may exist between the adenohypophysis and the hypothalamus, imposing additional regulation.

2.2 GROWTH HORMONE

Chemistry

Human growth hormone (HGH) has been purified and its amino acid sequence determined. It has a molecular weight of 21,500, and contains 188 amino acid residues and 2 disulfide bridges (Figure 2.4). A comparison of HGH with the purified growth hormones of seven other species is shown in Table 2.3. Although the molecular weights of growth hormones vary from 21,500 to 47,800, the heavier proteins may represent polymers having a unit molecular weight of 22,000. C. H. Li has suggested that bovine growth hormone (BGH) has a molecular weight of 45,000 and is composed of two chains with one C-terminal and two N-terminal amino acids and four disulfide bridges. Tryptic digestion of BGH results in a preparation that is metabolically active in humans and immunochemically reactive with rabbit anti-human growth hormone. The molecular weight of purified tryptic BGH is

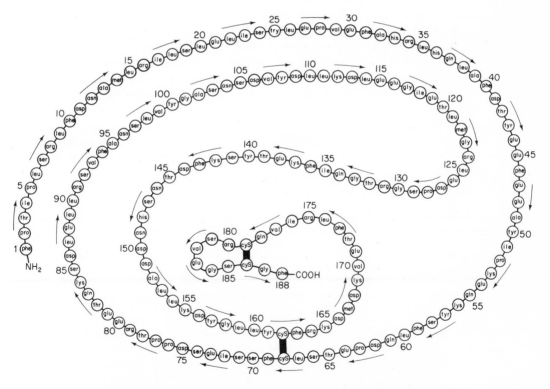

Figure 2.4 The amino acid sequence of human growth hormone (HGH). For names of the amino acids, see Appendix, page 155. All amino acids are here given in the *L* form. [From C. H. Li, "Current Concepts in the Chemical Biology of Pituitary Hormones." *Perspectives Biol. Med.,* 11, 498 (1968). Copyright © 1968 by the University of Chicago Press.]

approximately 22,000; some components of tryptic BGH have electrophoretic mobilities similar to HGH and several laboratories have reported molecular weights of 22,000 for BGH.

Growth hormones stimulate formation of specific antibodies; their immuno-chemical reactions with the sera produced by these antibodies have become a basis for hormonal assay. Similarity of structure among the growth hormones is indicated by the broad cross reactivity that exists between the hormones of various species and the antisera to growth hormones; for example, antiserum to rat or rabbit GH gives a precipitin reaction with GH prepared from rabbits, cattle, sheep, and pigs but no cross reaction with human or monkey GH.

Regulation of Secretion

The factors controlling the secretion of GH by the pituitary are unusually complex. Although it was known that lesions placed in the rat hypothalamus impaired growth and caused degranulation of acidophils in the adenohypophysis, the mechanism was not understood until hypothalamic hormonal control of adeno-hypophyseal function was recognized (Figure 2.5). The secretion of GH by the pituitary is increased by extracts from the hypothalamus; this observation was made first in vitro and later in vivo. Electrical stimulation of the ventromedial nucleus of the hypothalamus resulting in secretion of GH by the adenohypophysis has established this nucleus as one area that secretes GRH. Starvation causes a reduction of GH levels in the pituitary and GRH levels in the hypothalamus. Insulin causes a discharge of pituitary GH and administration of glucose blocks this discharge. a-2-Deoxy-D-glucose stimulates GH secretion and hyperglycemia; it causes a cellular glucopenia when converted to a-2-deoxy-D-glucose-6-phosphate,

TABLE 2.3 SOME PHYSIOCHEMICAL PROPERTIES OF GROWTH HORMONES
OBTAINED FROM PITUITARIES OF VARIOUS SPECIES[a]

Physiochemical Characteristics	Human	Monkey	Bovine[b]	Sheep	Pig	Whale	Rat	Rabbit
Molecular weight	21,500	23,000	45,000	47,800	41,600	39,900	46,000	46,000
Isoelectric point, pH	4.9	5.5	6.8	6.8	6.3	6.2	—	—
Sedimentation coefficient $S_{20,w}$	2.18	1.88	3.19	2.76	3.02	2.84	3.21[+c]	3.21[+c]
$[a]_d^{25°}$ (0.1 M HAc)	-39°	-55°	-36°	-49°	-47°	-52°	—	—
Diffusion coefficient, $D_{20} \times 10^7$	8.88	7.20	7.23	5.25	6.54	6.56	—	—
$-S-S-$ linkages	2	4	4	5	3	3	—	—
NH_2 -terminal amino acid	Phe	Phe	Phe,Ala	Phe,Ala	Phe	Phe	Phe	Phe
COOH - terminal amino acid	Phe	Phe	Phe	Phe	Phe	Phe	—	Phe

[a] Modified from C. H. Li, *Perspectives Biol. Med.*, **11**, 496, (1968).

[b] Monomer molecular weights of 22,000 have been suggested for bovine GH and may be applicable to other growth hormones that appear in approximate multiples of the monomer molecular weight.

[c] These values represent S_{20} buffer determined at pH 9.92 in 0.1 M H_3BO_3, 0.09 M NaOH and 0.15 M NaCl. When determined at pH 3.55 in 0.1 M glycine and 0.007 M HCl the S_{20} buffer was 2.24 and 1.44 respectively. S. Ellis, *et al, Ann. N.Y. Acad. Sci.*, **148**, 328, (1968).

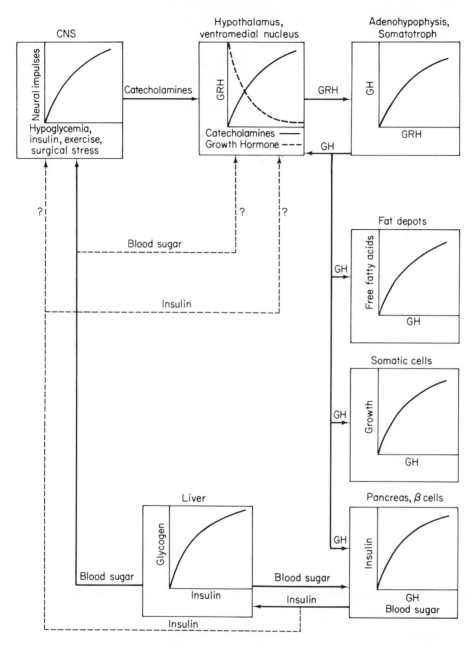

Figure 2.5 Control of GH secretion. Insulin and growth hormone are present in inverse concentrations in the plasma, and each can indirectly induce secretion of the other; this relationship may result in a positive-feedback control. The negative feedback may be due to the resulting concentration of plasma glucose. A further control may be a short negative-feedback loop created by GH inhibition of hypothalamic secretion of GRH. It is postulated that the control of secretion of GRH from the ventromedial nucleus is by release of catecholamines (norepinephrine and epinephrine L-dopamine), since drugs that inhibit α receptors or deplete cws catacholamine reserves (see Chapter 7) reduce the response to hypoglycemia and insulin.

which partially inhibits phosphoglucose isomerase and glucose-6-phosphate de-hydrogenase. Lesions in the hypothalamus block the increase in plasma GH levels that would otherwise be induced by insulin.

Insulin may induce GH release by causing a secretion of norepinephrine or L-dopamine. Drugs such as reserpine, a-methyl-dihydroxyphenylalanine (a-methyl-DOPA), a-methyl-m-tyrosine, or tetrabenazine cause depletion of norepinephrine reserves in the central nervous system and are able to prevent insulin-induced release of GH from the pituitary (Figure 2.5). Since in these experiments extreme hypoglycemias were induced, it is likely that the effect of low blood sugar levels on secretion of GH is also blocked by depletion of catecholamine (epinephrine or norepinephrine) stores in the central nervous system. Guanethidine and tyramine (depletors of peripheral norepinephrine stores) did not block the insulin-induced discharge of GH by the pituitary. The effect of insulin or reserpine on the concentration of GRH in the hypothalamus has also been examined: insulin causes and reserpine prevents depletion of hypothalamic stores of GRH. It is likely that the catecholamines may be the neurohumors involved in causing neurosecretory cells of the hypothalamus to release neurohormones. The induced secretion of insulin may complete the positive feedback control of GH secretion; both hormones are found in inverse concentrations in the plasma and each indirectly causes release of the other. A short loop between the pituitary and hypothalamus and the changing concentrations of glucose in the plasma may form the negative-feedback control.

Effect

The initial recognition of the pituitary's relationship to growth came from the correlation of gigantism, dwarfism, and acromegaly (due to hyperproduction of GH in the adult) with pathology of that gland. Evans first showed that BGH causes growth of young rats. The stimulatory action of GH on all major organs is most obvious in adult animals in which the visceral enlargement causes protrusion beyond the normal confines. Associated with growth is a markedly positive nitrogen balance; GH causes a reduction in plasma amino nitrogen, increases amino acid transport across cell membranes, and increases protein synthesis.

Growth hormone causes mobilization of nonesterified fatty acids from fat deposits while it also inhibits glucose utilization by muscle tissues and decreases the sensitivity of hypophysectomized animals to insulin. The first of these actions is the so-called ketogenic effect and the latter two are diabetogenic actions. Greater utilization of fat is also reflected by the respiratory quotient.

The development of sensitive radioimmunochemical assay techniques for highly purified pituitary hormones has made it possible to determine blood concentrations of these hormones in humans. The plasma concentration of GH in fasting human subjects is 1 to 2 ng/ml plasma; after exercise it rises to 17 to 53 ng/ml, reaching the highest point in the first hour of a 2-hr exercise period. Plasma free fatty acid concentrations also rise, while the blood glucose level remains constant. These changes are prevented if the subject ingests glucose. By making depot fat available, GH may play a role in providing cellular fuel, since fatty acids are metabolized only after they are mobilized from depots.

Current studies on GH action point to a role in the transcription or translation steps leading to protein biosynthesis. Widnell and Tata have shown an in vivo increase in liver ribonucleic acid (RNA) polymerase within 24 hr after GH treatment. Growth hormone has also been reported to stimulate transfer RNA (tRNA) and messenger RNA (mRNA) formation. Injection of GH into hypophysectomized rats can partially restore the lost ability of ribosomes to incorporate amino acids into proteins (Chapter 10).

2.3 THYROID-STIMULATING HORMONE

Chemistry

Thyroid-stimulating hormone (TSH) has not been prepared in pure form largely because of its instability and its formation of complexes with inert protein present in the preparation; TSH is also very difficult to separate from luteinizing hormone (LH), a contaminant in most preparations. The potency of the best preparations has varied from 20 to 200 IU*/mg. TSH is a glycoprotein having a molecular weight of about 28,000. The carbohydrate moiety, covalently bonded to a protein, appears to be a single oligosaccharide unit containing mannose, glucosamine, galactosamine, and fucose. Human TSH shows little cross reaction with bovine TSH antibodies prepared from rabbit serum, indicating immunochemical dissimilarities between the hormones of the different species.

Regulation of Secretion

Adenohypophyseal secretion of TSH is under dual control (Figure 2.6). There is evidence that thyroid hormone acts directly on the pituitary. Thyroid gland implants into the adenohypophyseal area of thyroidectomized rats retard the appearance of thyroidectomy cells among the thyrotrophs closest to the implants. Thyroxine (T_4) reduces the rate of ^{131}I release from the thyroids of hypophysectomized rabbits with implants of pituitary tissue in the anterior chamber of the eye. A dose of thyroxine so low that it causes no systemic effect, depresses ^{131}I rate of release from rabbit thyroid when instilled into the pituitary, but is ineffectual when injected into the hypothalamus. In organ culture of pituitaries, thyroxine reduces the secretion of TSH.

The existence of a hypothalamic feedback pathway is suggested by the isolation from the hypothalamus of a neurohormone (TRH) which induces the release of TSH. Other less direct evidence is that the thyroids of goitrogen (compounds causing enlargement of the thyroid) treated rats hypertrophy more than do the glands of rats given the same goitrogen but bearing bilateral hypothalamic lesions. In the latter case, the destroyed link in the chain is assumed to be the source of a substance regulating TSH secretion by the pituitary. The role of thyroid hormones

---

*The international unit (IU) is the amount of activity in 13.5 mg of International Standard Preparation. Assays must be performed with this material as the reference material.

in the regulation of TRH secretion is not fully established; a number of different stimuli are probably involved and the thyroid hormone may act through these stimuli by affecting caloric homeostasis (Figure 2.6).

Effects

Thyroid-stimulating hormone acts on two different sites: (1) the thyroid, and (2) the fat deposits, an extra-target site. In the latter, TSH induces release of fatty acids. Physiological levels of the hormone are sufficient for this lipolytic effect to be exerted.

The various actions of TSH on the thyroid have not been clearly differentiated. The first effect of TSH is an increased blood flow through the gland, and the second is an increase in the rate of breakdown of the colloid thyroglobulin. This proteolytic effect results in an increased thyroid hormone discharge and a reduced amount of colloid in the follicles. Simultaneously there is an increased biosynthesis of thyroid hormone, resulting in an increased rate of ^{131}I accumulation by the gland. A late consequence of TSH stimulation is an increase in size of the follicle cells and, when the stimulus is long-acting and intense, an increased number of cells and follicles.

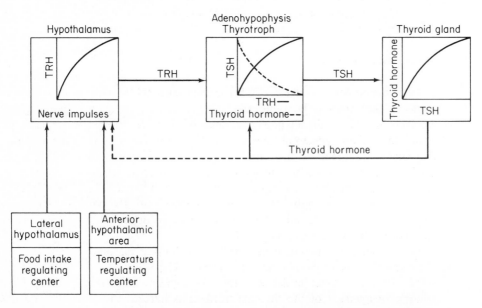

Figure 2.6   The regulation of thyroid-stimulating hormone (TSH) secretion occurs on two levels; one involves the direct interaction of thyroid hormones with the adenohypophysis and the second involves the hypothalamic control which is modulated by environmental and core temperatures, by food intake, and perhaps by the action of thyroid hormones on the hypothalamus. (TRH, thyroid-stimulating-hormone-releasing hormone.)

2.4 LONG-ACTING-THYROID STIMULATOR

In 1956 Adams and Purves described in the plasma of hyperthyroid patients a stimulatory substance which induced the discharge of organically bound ^{131}I from rat thyroid glands. Response to a dose of TSH required 2 to 3 hr while response to serum from hyperthyroid patients required 12 to 16 hr. Long-acting-thyroid stimulator (LATS) has been extracted from this serum and has been characterized as a 7-Svedberg (7-S)* ... a-globulin. It seems to be a specific a-globulin rather than an a-globulin-TSH complex. The molecule has been hydrolyzed to A and B chains with the A chain showing LATS activity. This substance is not present in the pituitary. LATS loses activity after incubation with minced thyroid tissues. Thus LATS may be an autoantibody against a thyroid component.

2.5 EXOPHTHALMOS-PRODUCING SUBSTANCE

Surgical intervention in the clinical condition of Graves disease is frequently followed by an exophthalmos (bulging of the eyes). Guinea pigs also show an exophthalmos after thyroidectomy. Although crude TSH preparations may induce exophthalmos, highly purified preparations do not. Many pituitary extracts and various subfractions have been examined; some have high concentrations of exophthalmos-producing substance and low levels of TSH activity, whereas others show the opposite condition. The consensus is that TSH and another hormone are involved; however, the exophthalmos factor has not yet been characterized.

2.6 ADRENOCORTICOTROPHIN

Chemistry

Adrenocorticotrophin (ACTH) is a single-chain polypeptide consisting of 39 amino acid residues and having a molecular weight of about 4,500 (see Figure 2.7); the ACTH molecule is the smallest of the adenohypophyseal hormones and has been completely characterized and synthesized. The hormone causes depletion of adrenal ascorbic acid and induces steroidogenesis. Similar effects can be elicited by a polypeptide consisting of the first 20 amino acids from the N-terminal end of the ACTH molecule. The amino acid sequences of ACTH of four species (pigs, cattle, sheep, and humans) have been determined. Species differences are confined to the amino acid residues numbered 25 through 33, and have no apparent effect on biological activity.

*Svedberg = a unit of time amounting to 10^{-13} sec that serves as a measure of the sedimentation velocity of a protein solution in an ultracentrifuge for use in determining the molecular weight of the protein.

ser-tyr-ser-met-glu-his-phe-arg-try-gly-lys-pro-val-gly-lys-lys-arg-arg-pro-val-lys-val-tyr-pro
 1   2   3   4   5   6   7   8   9 10 11 12 13 14 15 16 17 18 19 20 21 22 23 24

$$NH_2$$
Beef: asp-gly-glu-ala-glu-asp-ser-ala-glu-
         25 26 27 28 29 30 31 32 33

$$NH_2$$
Sheep: ala-gly-glu-asp-asp-glu-ala-ser-glu-   ala-phe-pro-leu-glu-phe
                                                  34 35 36 37 38 39

$$NH_2$$
Pig: asp-gly-ala-glu-asp-glu-leu-ala-glu-

Figure 2.7   The amino acid sequence of pig, sheep, and beef ACTH. For names of amino acids, see Appendix, page 155.

Regulation of Secretion

A number of diverse factors affect the adenohypophyseal secretion of ACTH. ACTH simultaneously inhibits the cellular secretion of CRH via a short negative-feedback loop and stimulates its target cells in the adrenal cortex. Furthermore, the cortical steroids in pharmacological doses may modify the activity of the adreno-cortical cells and in smaller dosage the cells that secrete CRH. Figure 2.8 summarizes the presently conceived pattern of regulation of ACTH secretion. Stress (any of a large variety of noxious stimuli) may provoke an increased secretion of ACTH, acting on the hypothalamus via central nervous system connections. Steroids implanted in the midbrain usually cause a reduction in adrenocortical secretion of corticosterone. This probably induces diffusely distributed steroid receptors to discharge, inhibiting the hypothalamic release of CRH. Hypothalamic extracts containing CRH have been shown to regulate ACTH secretion by the pituitary, and ACTH implanted into the hypothalamus has been shown to reduce the ACTH content of the adenohypophysis, probably due to the inhibition of neurosecretory-cell secretion of CRH. Glucocorticoids may have a direct action on the adenohypophyseal secretion of ACTH: they depress oxygen consumption of pituitary cultures and, when implanted into the vicinity of the pituitary, prevent the adrenal hypertrophy that occurs after unilateral adrenalectomy. Despite these indications of direct action of cortical steroids on the pituitary, the consensus is that the primary site of feedback action is the hypothalamus and perhaps other nervous areas. Vasopressin has also been shown to stimulate ACTH secretion but is not believed to be physiologically important.

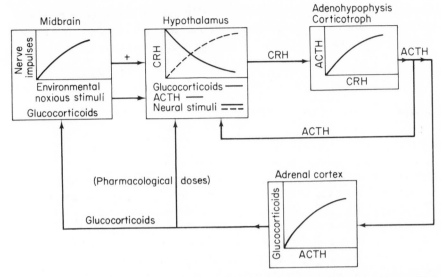

Figure 2.8 The regulation of adenohypophyseal secretion of adrenocorticotrophin by neural and hormonal stimuli. Particular note should be made of the dual neural control of the hypothalamus. The short negative-feedback loop between the adenohypophysis and hypothalamus is a novel control not often seen, but one which contributes an additional level of regulatory sensitivity. + or – indicates stimulation or inhibition, respectively.

Effects

Adrenocorticotrophin acts upon three sites. The targets that it primarily influences are the two innermost zones of cells in the adrenal cortex [the zona fasciculata and zona reticularis (see Chapter 7)]. These cell layers constitute the site of glucocorticoid synthesis and secretion. The zona glomerulosa (the outer cell layer of the cortex), which secretes aldosterone, is minimally affected by ACTH. The hormone also affects fat depots, where it exerts a lipolytic action in a manner similar to GH, TSH, and catecholamines. It stimulates melanocytes, causing darkening of skin in a manner similar to melanocyte-stimulating hormone (MSH).

The adrenal cortex is affected by ACTH in several ways: (1) It causes a reduction in the ascorbic acid content. (2) It concurrently converts cholesterol to glucocorticoids and increases their secretion rate. (3) It raises the level of metabolic activity of adrenal tissue through an increase in oxygen consumption and glucose utilization. (4) It stimulates cell division of the inner two layers and causes the cortex to grow. (5) It increases adenylcyclase activity and causes c-AMP synthesis with enhanced steroidogenesis proportionate to the ACTH dosage. Protein-synthesis inhibitors block the response to c-AMP but not the effect of ACTH on c-AMP concentration and glycogenolysis. The increased steroidogenesis may be due to increased conversion of cholesterol to pregnenolone (see Chapter 5).

2.7   PROLACTIN

Chemistry

Prolactin was among the first of the pituitary hormones to be prepared in almost pure form. The molecular weight of 23,000 pure ovine prolactin, calculated on the basis of sedimentation and diffusion, agrees with the result of amino acid analysis of 205 residues.

Human prolactin has all the properties of the best preparations of HGH and the two are indistinguishable by many criteria. However, the prolactin prepared from other species is distinct from their growth hormones.

Regulation of Secretion

There is evidence that the hypothalamus continually inhibits prolactin secretion by the adenohypophysis. Transplanted pituitary tissue continues to produce prolactin while the secretions of other hormones cease. Furthermore, cultured pituitary tissues release less prolactin to the medium when grown in a flask containing hypothalamic tissue than when grown alone; under similar conditions, more GH is formed and released when hypothalamic tissue is present. The hypothalamus is the source of a continuously secreted substance that inhibits prolactin release from the adenohypophysis. This substance is called prolactin-release-inhibiting hormone (PIH); see Figure 2.9.

Secretion of PIH is decreased in the lactating animal; termination of lactation has been associated with increased secretion of PIH. Therefore there should be an inverse relationship between amounts of prolactin and PIH secreted. Such a relationship has been observed and correlated with frequency of suckling by rat pups. As time of weaning approaches, the pups suckle less frequently and the prolactin content of the pituitary rises, reflecting the increased secretion of PIH.

The corpus luteum in the rat fails to function in the absence of prolactin, but this luteotrophic action of the hormone is seen only in rodents. Maintenance of a functional corpus luteum in rats is assumed, therefore, to be evidence of prolactin secretion. Estrogens, progesterone, and testosterone cause corpora lutea to continue functioning. Estrogen induces prolactin secretion by the pituitary; testosterone probably has a dual effect: (1) causing secretion of estrogen by the ovary, and (2) blocking neurosecretory-cell secretion of PIH. The progesterone effect is an example of a positive-feedback action, the pituitary production of prolactin is unaffected by large doses of the steroid (Figure 2.9).

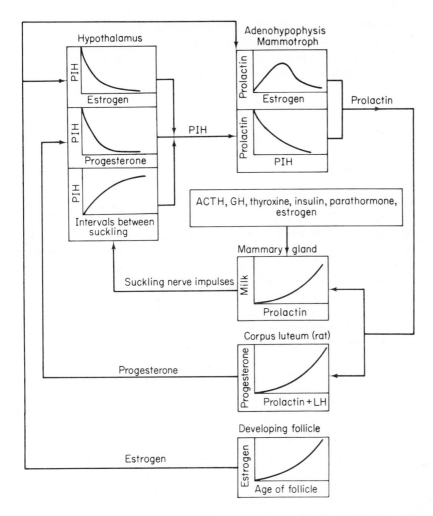

Figure 2.9   The regulation of the secretion of prolactin (mammotrophin or luteo-trophin). The problem of integrating control of lactation is compounded by the concurrent requirements for many other hormones. The secretion of prolactin is controlled by ovarian hormones that act on the hypothalamus and adenohypophysis, and by neural stimuli from the mammary gland. Prolactin entering into the median eminence blocks prolactin formation in the adenohypophysis by increasing PIH formation, which induces atrophy of mammary glands and cessation of lactation; estrogen depresses PIH formation.

Effects

It is apparent in nonmammalian vertebrates that prolactin has functions other than those of a lactogenic hormone. In pigeons, prolactin causes the crop sac to secrete "crop milk." In tadpoles the hormone inhibits tail resorption and urea excretion, and promotes growth after hypophysectomy. Prolactin stimulates a water drive in the land form of a newt (the red eft), and in some teleosts causes melanogenesis. In some euryhaline fish transferred to fresh water after hypophysectomy, administration of prolactin makes survival possible.

2.8 GONADOTROPHINS

Chemistry

Although no pure gonadotrophic hormones are available, five different preparations (three of nonpituitary origin) are currently in common use. Follicle-stimulating hormone (FSH) and LH are directly prepared from pituitary tissue. Human menopausal gonadotrophin (HMG), isolated from the urine of menopausal women, shows both FSH-like and LH-like activity. The serum from pregnant mares contains a gonadotrophin (PMS) which is predominantly FSH-like but with a small LH-like action. PMS is formed in the uterine endometrium and accumulates in the blood because it cannot be excreted by the kidney (see below). Human chorionic gonadotrophin (HCG) appears in the urine of women about 7 days after conception and reaches a peak in 6 wk. It exerts an LH-like effect, but FSH-like action appears with high doses.

The high glycosidic content of FSH and LH (Table 2.4) permits easy aqueous extraction from pituitary tissue. Ovine LH in acid solution dissociates into two nonidentical subunits with a molecular weight of about 15,000; in neutral or slightly alkaline solution, it has a molecular weight of 28,000 to 30,000. The two polypeptide subunits have different amino acid compositions. The LH molecule is believed to be a globular nonhelical molecule stabilized by cystine disulfide bridges. FSH contains 5 percent sialic acid which is essential for its activity, since neuraminidase digests this oligosaccharide and inactivates the hormone. HMG shows both FSH-like and LH-like activities, which tend to remain in the same ratio through purification procedures. This suggests a single molecule with dual actions. HCG derived from the placenta and PMS from the uterine endometrium are usually rich in carbohydrate, containing 30 and 50 percent, respectively. The high carbohydrate content may reflect contamination of these substances. The molecular weight of HCG is about 30,000, whereas that of PMS is 23,000. The apparent tendency of PMS to aggregate in electrolyte solutions may explain its failure to pass through renal membranes.

Regulation of Secretion

It is difficult to discuss one of the pituitary gonadotrophins, FSH or LH, without simultaneously considering the other, since functionally they complement each other. Spermatogenesis is possible only if both are secreted together, since FSH is needed in the intermediate stages of sperm development and interstitial-cell-

TABLE 2.4 CHEMICAL COMPOSITION OF GONADOTROPHIC HORMONES[a]

	Isoelectric Point	Molecular Weight	Nitrogen %	Carbohydrate %[c]	Number of Residues					Sialic Acid %	Cystine
					Glucosamine	Galactosamine	Mannose	Glucose	Fucose		
Luteinizing hormone (LH)	7.7	28,000	—	—	10	3	—	—	—	—	High
Follicle-stimulating hormone (FSH)	4.6	29,000	—	7.4	+	+	1.4	1.2	1.1	5	—
Human chorionic gonadotrophin (HCG)	2.95	30,000	10.5	19.7	12	3	9	—	2	8	—
Pregnant mare's serum gonadotrophin (PMS)	1.8	28,000	7.6	50.0	+	+	+	+	+	+	High
Human menopausal gonadotrophin (HMG)	—	31,000	—	30.0	—	—	—	—	—	8.5	—
Thyroid-stimulating hormone[b] (TSH)	—	28,000	—	7.9	6	3	9	—	1	1	High

[a]Modified from Goodman, L. S. and A. Gilman (eds.), *The Pharmacological Basis of Therapeutics,* 3rd ed. The Macmillan Company, New York, 1967.

[b] Thyroid-stimulating hormone is included because of its chemical similarity to the gonadrophins.

[c]Calculated on the basis of dry weight.

stimulating hormone (ICSH)* is needed to stimulate the androgen secretion necessary for sperm maturation. In the female, ovulation occurs only if both FSH and LH are sequentially available.

The negative-feedback loop in Figure 2.10 illustrates our current ideas on the regulation of gonadotrophin release in the male. The testosterone levels in the blood are thought to regulate activity of the neurosecretory cells that secrete the gonadotrophin-releasing hormones, FRH and LRH. Although the testes of some animals are rich sources of estrogens (for example, bull, stallion), the role of estrogens in male reproductive physiology and biochemistry is unknown. There is some evidence that the sex steroids directly affect the adenohypophysis; however, these pathways are not illustrated here.

Regulation of gonadotrophin secretion in the female is much more complicated than in the male (Figure 2.11). The secretion of both FSH and LH occurs at a constant basal level. In the human an intense surge of LH and FSH occurs on approximately the fourteenth day of the menstrual cycle. Rats maintained in animal rooms with light:dark cycles of 14 hr:10 hr and with the lights going on at 5:00 AM and off at 7:00 PM have 4 day cycles. In such rats FSH is probably released simultaneously with LH on the day of proestrus between 2:00 and 4:00 PM. Hilliard has shown that in the rabbit a positive-feedback system dependent on

*This name is given to "luteinizing hormone" when it is acting in the male.

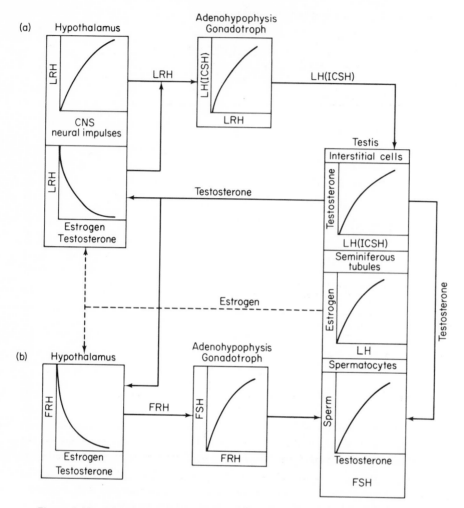

Figure 2.10 The regulation of gonadotrophin secretion in male mammals. The pathways in the upper part of the diagram (*a*) describe the regulation of LH secretion and the regulation of spermatogenesis by the resulting secretion of testosterone. (*b*) describes the regulation of FSH secretion and its action on the seminiferous tubule to contribute to spermatogenesis and perhaps to estrogen secretion. The dotted line indicates that it is not clear whether endogenous estrogens act in this manner.

the LH-stimulated secretion of 20α-hydroxypregn-4-en-3-one supports the secretion of LH until ovulation occurs.

Effects of Follicle-Stimulating Hormone

The role of FSH in males is unclear since FSH given in small doses to hypophysectomized rats does not maintain either the germinal epithelium or testicular weight. However, FSH and LH administered together in ratios of 4:1 to 400:1 do maintain testicular function. The combined action of these hormones probably

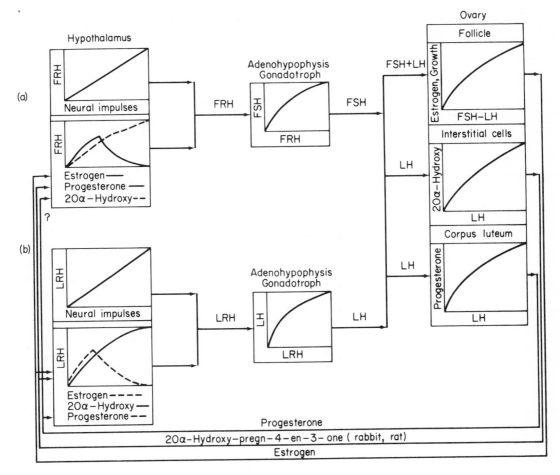

Figure 2.11 A generalized version of the regulation of the secretion of gonadotrophin in the female mammal (this scheme does not include an action of prolactin on the corpus luteum since this is specific to rodents). (*a*) FSH secretion by the pituitary gonadotrophic cells is determined by the hypothalamic secretion of FRH. It is assumed that all regulation of gonadotrophic-cell function is mediated via the hypothalamus. The control of hypothalamic function is dual; neural stimuli create a minimal level of function and hormones act as positive-feedback control at low concentrations. In higher concentrations these hormones become negative-feedback controls. Positive-feedback control intensifies the response and persists for a longer period than neural stimuli. (*b*) LH secretion is controlled by the adenohypophyseal gonadotrophic cells. This mechanism at present appears to be directly superimposable on the pattern for control of FSH secretion.

involves stimulation of androgen secretion as final maturation of the sperm requires the presence of androgens.

In females, FSH acts on growing follicles to stimulate their maturation. The transition from an immature oocyte surrounded by a single layer of granulosa cells to a mature structure involves stimulation of mitotic activity and consequent growth of three different cell types: (1) connective tissue cells that form the outer layers of follicles; (2) theca interna cells in the middle layer; and (3) granulosa cells in the innermost layer.

Effects of Luteinizing Hormone

In males, ICSH causes the interstitial cells to secrete testosterone. There is little evidence to indicate cyclic release of ICSH from the adenohypophysis, except in seasonal breeders, for example, deer. In animals such as rabbit, dog, rat, and man, there is continuous stimulation of the interstitial cells.

In females, ovulation may either occur spontaneously as part of a cycle, or as a reflex in response to a stimulus (most commonly coitus). Rats, dogs, sheep, and most primates are spontaneous ovulators, whereas cats, ferrets, and rabbits are reflexive. The action of LH is more easily understood in the latter group. The initial response of a rabbit to LH occurs within seconds of the secretion of the hormone and constitutes a hyperemic reaction, perhaps due to a local release of histamine. The next response appears within minutes and is manifested by discharge of a progestin (20α-hydroxypregn-4-en-3-one) from the interstitial cells. The mature follicle is noticeably enlarged 6 hr after coitus and ruptures after 10 to 11 hr. Following the rupture, the granulosa cells hypertrophy and increase their secretory activities and the entire follicular space becomes filled with large lipid-containing cells, becoming a corpus luteum (Chapter 6). Stimulation of steroid biosynthesis by ICSH (LH) in interstitial cells and the corpus luteum may involve the generation of c-AMP as a "second messenger" in a manner similar to the action of other hormones such as ACTH, TSH, vasopressin, and norepinephrine upon their targets (see Chapter 10).

2.9   THE LIPOTROPHINS

In 1936 Best and Campbell described a fat-mobilizing effect of anterior pituitary extracts. Subsequent preparations having specific lipotrophic effects were obtained, and in 1965 and 1966 Li and co-workers isolated two lipolytic polypeptides and determined their structures: one, with 90 amino acids and a molecular weight of 9,500, was designated β-lipotrophin (β-LPH); the second, with 58 amino acids and a molecular weight of 5,810, was named γ-lipotrophin (γ-LPH). The amino acid sequences are shown in Figure 2.12. The γ-LPH molecule is represented in its entirety in the β-LPH molecule. These lipolytic polypeptides, ACTH, and MSH all share a common heptapeptide core (Figure 2.13), which exhibits MSH-type activity (see section 2.10).

In vitro MSH activity of β-LPH is about twice as great as that of γ-LPH: the former has an activity of about 1.9×10^{11} units/mole and the latter about 0.9×10^{11} units/mole. The same two-to-one relationship of the two lipotrophins is true for in vitro lipolytic activity in rabbit adipose tissue. In the rat, sheep γ-LPH is inactive while β-LPH is active at concentrations 10 to 50 times higher than in the rabbit by the lipolytic assay performed on adipose tissues of the two species.

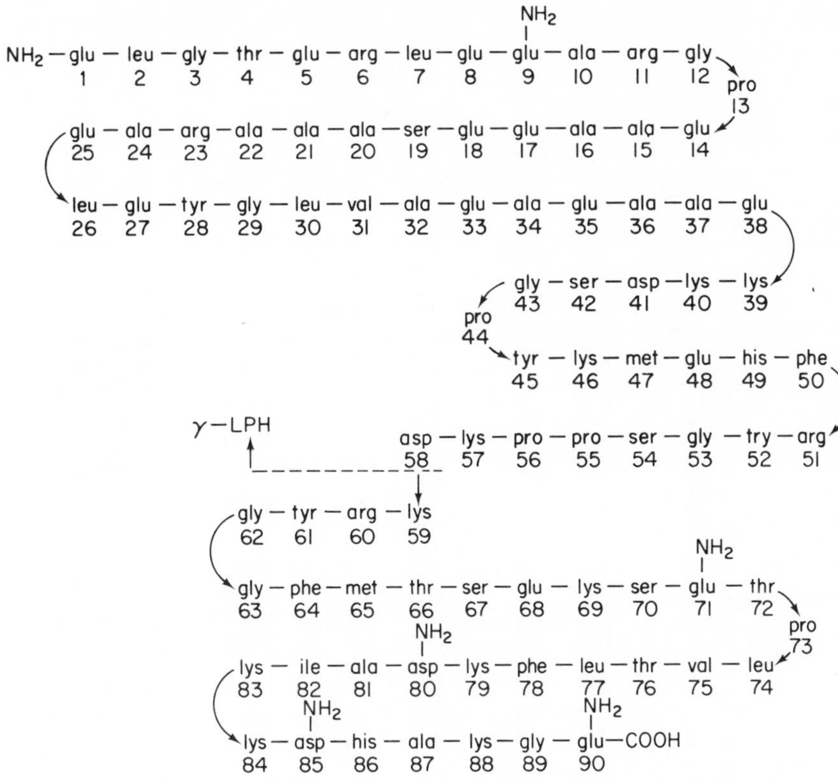

Figure 2.12 The amino acid sequence of sheep β-lipotrophin (β-LPH) is represented by the sequence 1 through 90. The sequence 1 through 58 represents γ-LPH. These substances are lipolytic and melanotrophic, and both possess a small amount of adrenocorticotrophic activity. [From C. H. Li, "Current Concepts on the Chemical Biology of Pituitary Hormones," *Perspectives Biol. Med.*, **11**, 498 (1968). Copyright ©1968 by the University of Chicago Press.]

Little is known about the regulation of secretion of the lipotrophic hormones or the role they play in the vertebrate organism.

2.10 MELANOCYTE-STIMULATING HORMONE

Chemistry

Melanocyte-stimulating hormone (MSH) has been demonstrated to be in the anterior lobe of the pituitary of all vertebrates and in the intermediate lobe of those vertebrates possessing such a structure. It is present in mammalian pituitaries in two forms designated by Lerner as α- and β-MSH. The former, a tridecapeptide, has greater biological activity and has been found in all mammals; β-MSH has a variable chain length (the human hormone has 22 amino acids, whereas β-MSH in pigs, cattle, and horses has 18) and amino acid sequence. All the MSH molecules have a

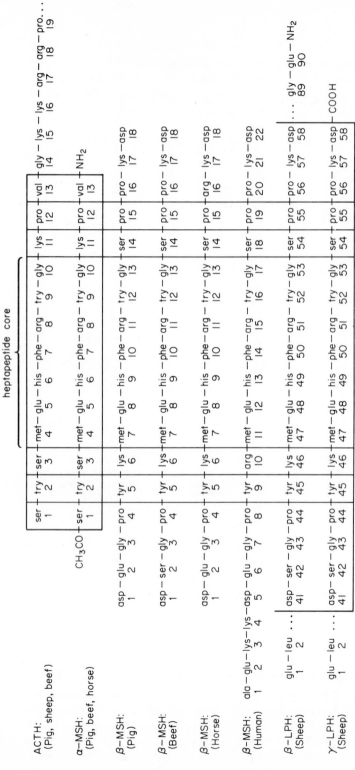

Figure 2.13 The relationships among the structure of melanotrophins (MSH), the partial structure of adrenocorticotrophic hormone (ACTH), and β- and γ-LPH. [From J. S. Dixon and C. H. Li, "The Isolation and Structure of β-Melanocyte-Stimulating Hormone from Horse Pituitary Glands," *Gen. Comp. Endocrinol.*, 1, 161–169 (1961), and C. H. Li, "Current Concepts on the Chemical Biology of Pituitary Hormones," *Perspectives Biol. Med.*, 11, 498 (1968).]

common heptapeptide core, which is also contained in ACTH and β- and γ-lipotrophin (Figure 2.13). Furthermore, a-MSH has a sequence of 13 amino acids identical to that at the N-terminal end of ACTH. However, the N-terminal seryl residue of a-MSH is acetylated, that of ACTH is not. The C-terminal valyl residue of a-MSH is in the amide form, while the corresponding valyl of ACTH connects to a continuing amino acid sequence.

Human β-MSH and bovine β-MSH have been synthesized and relationships between structure and activity have been explored. The heptapeptide core, met-glu-his-phe-arg-try-gly, has melanophore-dispersing activity, but the smallest sequence still possessing such activity is the pentapeptide, his-phe-arg-try-gly. Maximum activity is attained with the tridecapeptide sequence found in N-terminal-acetylated a-MSH (Table 2.5).

TABLE 2.5 MELANOCYTE-STIMULATING ACTIVITY
OF SYNTHETIC PEPTIDES[a]

Peptide	MSH Activity (units/gm)
H-ser-tyr-ser-met-glu-his-phe-arg-try-gly-lys-pro-val-gly-lys-lys-arg-arg-pro-OH 1 2 3 4 5 6 7 8 9 10 11 12 13 14 15 16 17 18 19	1.4×10^7
H$_3$CO-ser-tyr-ser-met-glu-his-phe-arg-try-gly-lys-pro-val-NH$_2$ 1 2 3 4 5 6 7 8 9 10 11 12 13	3.3×10^{10}
NH$_2$ | H-ser-try-ser-met-glu-his-phe-arg-OH 1 2 3 4 6 7 8	—
NH$_2$ | H-ser-met-glu-his-phe-arg-try-gly-OH 3 4 6 7 8 9 10	7×10^5
Tosyl | H-his-phe-arg-try-gly-lys-pro-val-NH$_2$ 6 7 8 9 10 11 12 13	5×10^5
NH$_2$ | H-met-glu-his-phe-arg-OH 4 6 7 8	—
H-his-phe-arg-try-gly-OH 6 7 8 9 10	$1.5–3 \times 10^4$
H-glu-his-phe-arg-try-gly-OH 5 6 7 8 9 10	2.2×10^5
H-met-glu-his-phe-arg-try-gly-OH 4 5 6 7 8 9 10	1.4×10^6

[a]Modified from H. Papkoff, and C. H. Li, "Hormone Structure and Biological Activity: Biochemical Studies of Three Pituitary Hormones," Table 9, *J. Chem. Educ.* **43**, 41 (1966).

Regulation of Secretion

The dispersion of pigment in the frog skin is caused by MSH; concentration of pigment may be controlled by melatonin, produced by the pineal gland (Chapter 9). Figure 2.14 illustrates the presently conceived regulation of MSH secretion as being dependent on the release of an MSH-release-inhibiting hormone (MIH), produced in the supraoptic region of the hypothalamus. Melatonin may act on the hypothalamus to stimulate secretion of MIH and directly on the melanophore to cause pigment concentration around the nucleus and blanching of the skin.

Effects

Melanin-containing cells are generally of two types. In cold-blooded vertebrates, melanin is contained in *melanophores.* Skin color is determined by the distribution of pigment in the cytoplasm; the skin is pale when the pigment is concentrated near the nucleus and dark when widely dispersed through the cytoplasm of the cell. In birds and mammals, melanin is contained in *melanocytes.* These cells synthesize and store their pigment, and can contribute it to adjacent cells and structures. The α-MSH causes increased synthesis of melanin in both melanophores and melanocytes and dispersion of melanin in melanophores. The role of α-MSH and β-MSH in mammals is not clear. In cold-blooded vertebrates— fish, amphibia, and reptiles—α-MSH serves a protective function; the animal becomes pale on a light background and dark on a dark background. Adrenocorticotrophin can also cause darkening of the skin (bronzing of the skin in Addison's disease) in a manner similar to that of α-MSH.

The α-MSH exerts a thyrotrophic action on thyroid tissue and both α- and β-MSH cause an increased lipolysis of adipose tissue in vitro. These effects may not be physiologically important.

2.11   THE NEUROHYPOPHYSEAL HORMONES

The secretions associated with the neurohypophysis are produced in the hypothalamus. Seven natural cyclic nonapeptides have been identified in vertebrate neurohypophyseal extracts (Figure 2.15): oxytocin, vasotocin, mesotocin, ichthyotocin (isotocin), glumitocin, arginine vasopressin, and lysine vasopressin. In reptiles, birds, and mammals, these secretions originate in the supraoptic and paraventricular nuclei, while in fish and amphibia they originate in the preoptic nuclei. The hormones are transmitted through the axons of the neurons that compose these nuclei to the capillary beds in the neurohypophysis. There the hormones are stored in granules accumulated at the axon terminals; they must be released from these granules (neurophysins) before they can be secreted. The neurophysins may be involved in transport and storage of the hormones. Three hormone-binding proteins, neurophysin I, II, and III, have been isolated. Neurophysin III appears in smaller amounts than either I or II. The mechanism that causes hormone release is

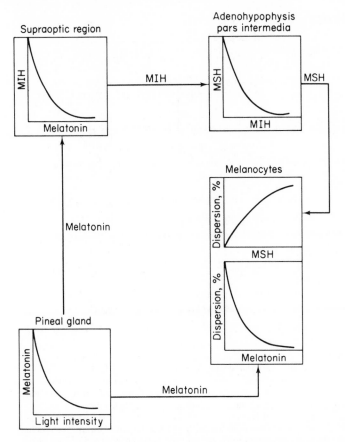

Figure 2.14 Control of melanocyte-stimulating hormone (MSH) secretion. No feedback from the periphery is seen. Concentration of pigment by melanocyte cells is also possible by the direct action of catecholamines on these cells. MSH-release-inhibiting hormone (MIH) is the major regulator of MSH secretion. The pineal gland probably plays an important role in melanocyte function in amphibians; in higher vertebrates, the pineal gland exerts control on the secretion of gonadotrophin.

not known; the axon terminals may abut on either the basement membranes of capillaries or cells surrounding the capillaries. In mammals, each hormone is secreted independently from its own hypothalamic nucleus; the supraoptic nucleus has been associated with vasopressin secretion and the paraventricular nucleus with oxytocin secretion.

Chemistry

Oxytocin and arginine vasopressin are present in the posterior pituitaries of all mammals except the hog, which has lysine vasopressin. Oxytocin and arginine vasotocin are found in birds, reptiles, and some amphibians; vasotocin and ichthyotocin (isotocin) are found in some teleost fish. Mesotocin has been isolated

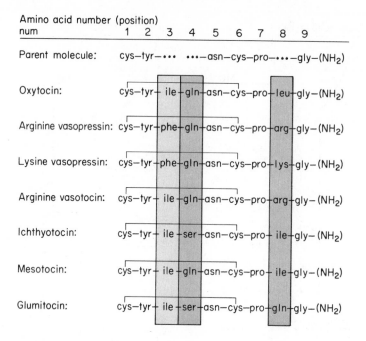

Amino acid number (position)

| num | | 1 | 2 | 3 | 4 | 5 | 6 | 7 | 8 | 9 |

Parent molecule: cys—tyr—••• •••—asn—cys—pro—•••—gly—(NH₂)

Oxytocin: cys—tyr—ile—gln—asn—cys—pro—leu—gly—(NH₂)

Arginine vasopressin: cys—tyr—phe—gln—asn—cys—pro—arg—gly—(NH₂)

Lysine vasopressin: cys—tyr—phe—gln—asn—cys—pro—lys—gly—(NH₂)

Arginine vasotocin: cys—tyr—ile—gln—asn—cys—pro—arg—gly—(NH₂)

Ichthyotocin: cys—tyr—ile—ser—asn—cys—pro—ile—gly—(NH₂)

Mesotocin: cys—tyr—ile—gln—asn—cys—pro—ile—gly—(NH₂)

Glumitocin: cys—tyr—ile—ser—asn—cys—pro—gln—gly—(NH₂)

Figure 2.15   The molecular structure of the seven known natural neurohypophyseal hormones and the probable parent molecule from which they originated. One gene duplication and a series of subsequent single substitutions in position 3, 4, or 8 could produce two molecular "lines." Thus substitution of isoleucine for glutamine in position 8 transforms glumitocin into ichthyotocin, and substitution of glutamine for serine in position 4 transforms ichthyotocin into mesotocin. The mammalian hormone oxytocin appears with the substitution of leucine for arginine in position 8 of vasotocin. Arginine vasopressin appears by the substitution of phenylalamine for ichthyotocin in position 3 of vasotocin.

from the posterior pituitary of some amphibians and lungfish and may be present in reptiles. Glumitocin has been identified in cartilaginous fish (rayfish and dogfish) and prepared from the neurohypophyses of rayfish (Table 2.6). All the hormones contain a pentapeptide ring joined by a disulfide bond between two half-cystine molecules at the 1 and 6 positions. This ring structure containing 20 atoms is essential to biological activity. The hormones differ in amino acid composition at the 3, 4, and 8 positions. The amino acids at the 1, 2, 5, 6, 7, and 9 positions are constant in the hormones presently known.

These hormones have similar qualitative activities, but they differ remarkably in their quantitative effects (Table 2.7). As an antidiuretic in the amphibian assay, arginine vasotocin (3-ile, 8-arg) is approximately 400 times as effective as arginine vasopressin (3-phe, 8-arg). In rat antidiuresis assays, arginine vasopressin is about twice as active as lysine vasopressin. In the rabbit milk ejection assay, oxytocin (3-ile, 8-leu) is about eight times as effective as either arginine vasopressin or lysine vasopressin, whereas in the rat uterus assay oxytocin is four times as effective as the

TABLE 2.6 PHYLOGENETIC DISTRIBUTION OF THE NEURO-
HYPOPHYSEAL HORMONES

Class	Oxytocin Principle	Vasopressin Principle
Mammalia	Oxytocin	Arginine vasopressin[a]
Aves	Oxytocin	Arginine vasotocin
Reptilia	Mesotocin	Arginine vasotocin (chromatographic and pharmacologic evidence only)
Amphibia	Mesotocin	Arginine vasotocin
Pisces		
Teleosts	Isotocin	Arginine vasotocin
Ray-finned fish	Glumitocin	Arginine vasotocin (?)
Lungfish	Mesotocin (perhaps oxytocin also)	Arginine vasotocin
Cyclostones	—	Arginine vasotocin

[a] An exception is the hog, which has lysine vasopressin.

8-lysyl analogs. Glumitocin shows a low level of oxytocin activity which is increased tenfold in the presence of magnesium ions.

Oxytocin is most active when the 3 and 8 positions are filled by isoleucine and leucine, respectively. Substitutions of other amino acids uniformly reduce oxytocin activity, more for uterine contraction than for milk ejection. Antidiuresis in rats is most effective when the side chain contains a basic amino acid such as arginine; the effect is decreased when lysine is substituted and even further decreased when citrulline is substituted for arginine.

Regulation of Vasopressin Secretion

Regulation of vasopressin (antidiuretic hormone) secretion may be initiated by a number of different pathways converging on the hypothalamus (Figure 2.16). Alteration of plasma osmotic pressure is probably the primary regulatory mechanism; however, alteration of blood volume or blood pressure, which activates volume receptors in the right atrium or baroceptors of the carotid arteries, also contributes to the control of vasopressin secretion. An increase in blood volume and consequent distention of the right atrium causes a diuresis, while hemorrhage, when accompanied by a reduced blood volume and pressure, causes water reten-

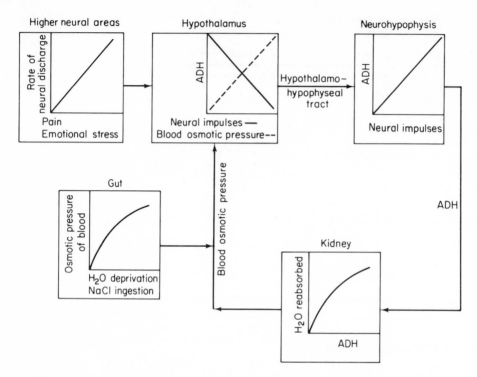

Figure 2.16 Control of water reabsorption by vasopressin acting as the antidiuretic hormone (ADH). Although plasma osmolality is probably the primary regulator, other factors may contribute to the regulation of the excretion of water.

tion. Extrinsic factors such as pain, which affect the nervous system, induce an emotional stress inhibiting the secretion of vasopressin.

Regulation of Oxytocin Secretion

Although oxytocin has no demonstrated role in males, it has a well-established role in females. In pregnant animals parturition can be induced and brought to completion with oxytocin. During parturition the plasma oxytocin in cows increases from 55 μU/ml (microunits per milliliter) in the first stage of labor to between 10 and 20 times this amount during the second stage, and falls to control levels 2 hr after delivery. In second-stage labor in women, there is a threefold increase in plasma oxytocin concentration (from 50 to 150 μU/ml). Oxytocin release is inhibited by progesterone in rats, rabbits, pigs, and cows, but not in sheep or women.

Oxytocin also is important in the lactating female since in its absence no milk is released from the mammary gland. Ejection of milk occurs after administration of

TABLE 2.7 COMPARISON OF THE ACTIVITIES OF THE NEUROHYPOPHYSEAL HORMONES[a,b]

	Molecular Weight	(1) Isolated Rat Uterus	(2) Chicken Blood Pressure	(3) Rabbit Mammary Gland	(4) Rat Anti-Diuresis	(5) Rat Blood Pressure
Oxytocin	1007.2	450	450	450	5	5
Ichthyotocin (ser^4-ile^8-oxytocin)	966.2	150	320	300	0.18	0.06
Arginine vasopressin (phe^3-arg^8-oxytocin)	1084.2	16	60	65	400	400
Lysine vasopressin (ile^3-lys^8-oxytocin)	1056.2	5	40	60	250	270
Arginine vasotocin (arg^8-oxytocin)	1050.2	115	285	210	250	245
Mesotocin (ile^8-oxytocin)	1007.2	291	502	330	1.1	6.3
Glumitocin (ser^4-glu^8-oxytocin)	981.1	8	—	—	—	—

[a]Data modified from B. Berde and R. A. Boissannas, "Neurohypophyseal Hormones and Similar Polypeptides," in B. Berde (ed.), *Handbuch der experimentellen Pharmokologie,* vol. 23, Springer-Verlag, Berlin and New York, 1968. All activities here are expressed in international units/μmole. The international unit for oxytocin and vasopressin is the amount of pituitary hormone contained in 0.5 mg of acetone-dried posterior pituitary powder. One milligram of pure synthetic oxytocin has an activity of 450 IU, or 1 IU of oxytocic potency is contained in 2.2 μg of synthetic oxytocin. One milligram of synthetic arg^8 vasopressin has a pressor potency of 400 IU, or 1 IU represents either pressor or antidiuretic potency of 2.5 μg of arg^8 vasopressin. All assays are based on these standards.

[b]Bioassay procedures used are as follows: (1) The *isolated rat-uterus assay* is based on the enhanced contractility of uterine smooth muscle. The uterus is obtained from estrus-stage rats or rats treated with estrogen for 3 successive days. The contractility of the uterus in a bath 28 to $30°C$ is determined with administration of hormone (standard and unknown). (2) The *chicken blood pressure assay* is measured with the ischiatric artery cannulated; the decrease in pressure resulting from treatment with oxytocic standard and unknown is determined. (3) The *rabbit mammary gland* milk duct is cannulated and the volume or pressure response to intravenous injection of an oxytocic standard and unknown is determined. (4) The *rat-antidiuresis assay* is based on the ability of vasopressin standard and the unknown to reduce the rate of formation of urine in hydrated rats. (5) The *rat blood pressure* assay is determined by measuring the elevation of blood pressure in response to doses of hormone (standard and unknown).

oxytocin or after the application of an electrical stimulus to the paraventricular nucleus, infundibulum, or any point on the hypothalamohypophyseal tract. Secretion of oxytocin can be prevented by anesthetizing the suckled teat, cutting the innervation of the gland, placing lesions in the paraventricular nucleus, or sectioning the pituitary stalk (Figure 2.17).

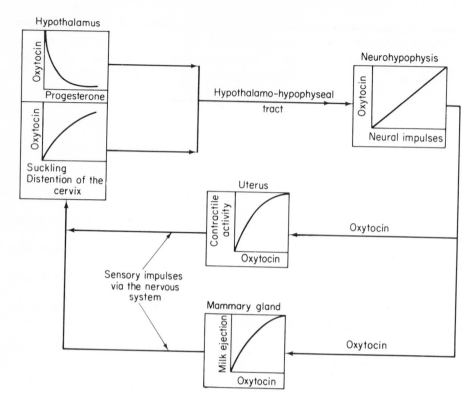

Figure 2.17   Control of oxytocin secretion in the pregnant and lactating animal. In some mammals, the decline in the secretion of progesterone with aging of the placenta causes a secretion of oxytocin, which induces parturition. Once initiated, the process becomes a positive-feedback system, since distention of the cervix induces further secretion of oxytocin. The relationship of suckling to oxytocin is that of a positive-feedback system.

Effects of Vasopressin and Oxytocin

These hormones are capable of causing similar responses of different magnitudes (Table 2.7). In physiological doses, vasopressin exerts an antidiuretic effect; in larger doses, it causes contraction of smooth muscle, especially in the blood vessels. At present, oxytocin is thought to be important only in the pregnant and lactating female, where it causes contraction of the uterine muscle and ejection of milk. The mechanism by which it acts on smooth muscle cells is not known; however, the speed of this response is thought to be due to a membrane-dependent phenomenon.

Vasopressin manifests its action largely by affecting water and urea permeability of renal nephrons, and frog and toad bladders. The absence of vasopressin in mammals results in diabetes insipidus, a condition in which large volumes of water are consumed and then lost in the urine. The most acceptable hypothesis to explain the action of vasopressin (and perhaps oxytocin) was proposed by Orloff and Handler, who suggested that the hormone triggers the activity of the adenyl cyclase system in cell membranes. This proposal is based on the observation that vasopressin increases concentrations of c-AMP in susceptible tissues (c-AMP induces effects similar to vasopressin as does theophylline, which protects c-AMP against destruction by phosphodiesterase).

REFERENCES ――――――――――――――――――――――――――――――

Bell, E. T.: "Some Observations on the Assay of Anterior Pituitary Hormones," *Vitamins and Hormones*, **24**, 63-113 (1966).

Berde, B., and R. A. Boissannas: "Neurohypophyseal Hormones and Similar Polypeptides," in B. Berde (ed.), *Handbuch der experimentellen Pharmakologie*, vol. 23, Springer-Verlag, Berlin and New York, 1961.

Harris, G. W., and B. T. Donovan: *The Pituitary*, vol. 3, University of California Press, Berkeley, 1966.

Martini, L., and W. F. Ganong: *Neuroendocrinology*, vol. 2, Academic Press, New York, 1966.

Pincus, G., K. V. Thiman, and E. B. Astwood (eds.): *The Hormones*, vol. 5, Academic Press, New York, 1964.

Ramachandran, J., and Chah-Hao Li: "Structure-Activity Relationships of the Adrenocorticotropins and Melanotropins: The Synthetic Approach," *Adv. Enzymol.*, **29**, 391-479 (1967).

THREE | THYROXINE AND TRIIODOTHYRONINE

The thyroid gland is the source of two different kinds of hormones. The best known is a group constituting a unique category of substances, the iodinated derivatives of thyronine. The second is a recently discovered polypeptide, calcitonin, which is involved in the regulation of calcium levels in the blood (see Chapter 8).

The thyroid gland utilizes iodine, the heaviest element found in living systems, in the biosynthesis of the thyronines. This synthesis is the only example of an authentic biological requirement for a halogen atom. The treatment of goiters with an essential trace component found in burnt kelp has been known since ancient times. The presence of iodine in the thyroid gland, however, was not firmly established until 1895 by Baumann. The recognition of thyroglobulin as a principal storage form of iodine by Oswald followed in 1899. The isolation of thyroxine by E. C. Kendall in 1914 ultimately led to the elucidation of its structure and its synthesis by C. R. Harington of England in 1927. Since then, seven other iodinated amino acids have been isolated and identified as constituents of the normal thyroid gland (Table 3.1). However, the designation of "thyroid hormone" is generally limited to L-3,5,3'-triiodothyronine (T_3) and/or L-thyroxine (T_4).

TABLE 3.1 ORGANIC IODINE COMPOUNDS OF THE
THYROID GLAND

L-Amino Acid	When Identified	Total Iodine in Human Thyroid,%	Relative Biological Activity (Rat)
Thyroxine (T$_4$)[a]	1915	35±5	1.0
3,5-Diiodotyrosine (DIT)	1929	30±5	<0.01
3-Monoiodotyrosine (MIT)	1948	20±5	0
3,5,3'-Triiodothyronine (T$_3$)	1952	5±2	5.0
3,3'5'-Triiodothyronine	1956	Trace	0.05
3,3'-Diiodothyronine	1956	Trace	0.2
Monoiodohistidine	1952	Trace	0
Diiodohistidine	1958	Trace	0

[a]Thyroxine is 3,5,3',5'-tetraiodothyronine. The primed numbers
refer to substituents on ring B.

The structure of thyronine is:

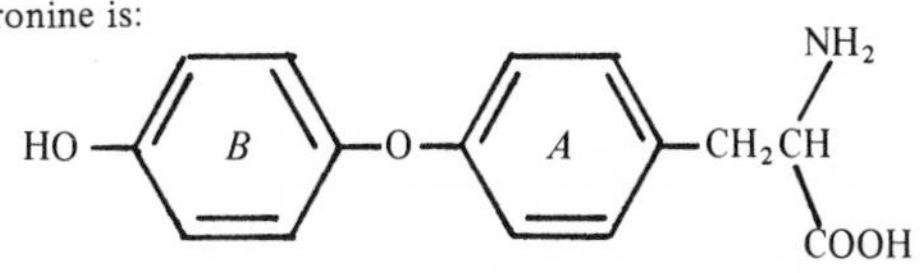

In many vertebrates the thyroid gland consists of two lobes, sometimes connected by a narrow isthmus across the ventral surface of the trachea. In the human, the normal gland weighs 30 ± 10 g; the dimensions of each lobe are 4 × 2.5 × 2 cm. The thyroid is composed mainly of spherical follicles dispersed in a highly vascularized tissue matrix. Each follicle consists of a single peripheral layer of medium or low cuboidal epithelial cells enclosing a colloidal aggregation of thyroglobulin. The size of the follicle is determined by the functional state of the gland, which in turn is established by the concentration of TSH in the blood. Thyroid enlargement, giving rise to goiter, is due to excessive stimulation of the thyroid by TSH. Excessive TSH production may be caused by inadequate production of T$_3$ or T$_4$ (due to a dietary iodine deficiency), by poor iodide absorption, or by excessive production of TSH (due to a failure in pituitary regulation). With excessive TSH production, the enlarged thyroid secretes large amounts of T$_3$ and T$_4$; the most prominent effect of this is a hyperthyroid state (see Figure 2.6). The long-acting thyroid stimulator (LATS), an abnormal protein found in the plasma, may also cause a hyperthyroid state. In regions where there is inadequate dietary iodine, goiter appears in an endemic form. It was initially recognized in a population of school children, and was quickly cured by dietary supplementation with iodine. The goiter produced by iodine deficiency is characterized by large follicles filled with a colloid-like material; the cells of the follicle linings are very short (squamous) or cuboidal. The goiter caused by excessive TSH secretion is characterized by small follicles containing little colloid and lined with columnar epithelial cells.

3.1 IODINE METABOLISM AND THE BIOSYNTHESIS OF THYROID HORMONES

The biosynthesis of the principal naturally occurring active thyroid hormones, T_4 and T_3, is closely related to the special metabolism of inorganic and organic iodides (Figure 3.1). Dietary iodide, absorbed as inorganic iodide, is removed from the plasma and concentrated by the thyroid gland. This "halogen-pumping mechanism" can be saturated by an excess of iodide; however, it is dependent on thyroid gland activity, which is regulated by pituitary secretion. The accumulation of iodide prior to its incorporation into the phenyl ring of the hormone is stimulated by TSH and blocked by thiocyanate (SCN^-) and perchlorate (ClO_4^-). The active biosynthesis of thyroid hormones proceeds through a series of steps beginning with the formation of "active molecular iodine (I_2)" by a peroxidase, a process which is inhibited by the antithyroid SH-containing goitrogens (for example, 2-thiouracil and thiourea, Figure 3.2). The active I_2 then selectively iodinates tyrosyl molecules of the polypeptides which subsequently give rise to thyroglobulin. The iodination products are 3-monoiodotyrosine (MIT), 3,5-diiodotyrosine (DIT), and finally the various combinations of their oxidative condensation products: mostly T_4, some T_3, and traces of 3,3'-diiodothyronine and 3,3',5-triiodothyronine (see Table 3.1). Both the formation of organic iodine compounds and the coupling reaction appear to be blocked by a variety of synthetic and a few natural goitrogenic agents. These include thiourea, sulfaguanidine, propylthiouracil, 2-mercaptoimidazole, and several naturally occurring compounds: 5-vinyl-2-thiooxazolidone (yellow turnips) and

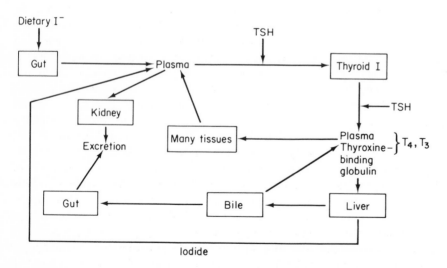

Figure 3.1 The metabolism of inorganic and organic iodine in the mammal, emphasizing the central role of the plasma iodide. An important aspect of the metabolism of iodine involves the enterohepatic recyling of thyroid hormone from intestine to liver, (TBG, thyroxine-binding globulin.)

allylthiourea (mustard). The best available explanation for this action is that the goitrogenic agents inhibit the action of peroxidases necessary for the production of active I_2 and poison the free-radical milieu required for the coupling reaction. The ability of these agents to produce goiters is illustrated by the fact that when given to rats in their drinking water (0.010 percent), 6-*n*-propyl-2-thiouracil will produce a goiter in 7 to 10 days weighing 55 mg/100 g body weight from an initial gland of less than 10 mg/100 g body weight.

The coupling reaction in which two substituted phenols are condensed to the corresponding diphenyl ether is depicted in Figure 3.3. This unusual chemical transformation has attracted the continuing interest of organic chemists and has been studied in model systems in which DIT and its derivatives are converted to the corresponding T_4 derivative in good yield. The best yields are obtained when DIT is condensed with 3,5-diiodo-4-hydroxyphenylpyruvic acid to yield T_4 and pyruvate, or when two molecules of *N*-acetyl-3,5-diiodotyrosyl-*N*-acetyllysine are

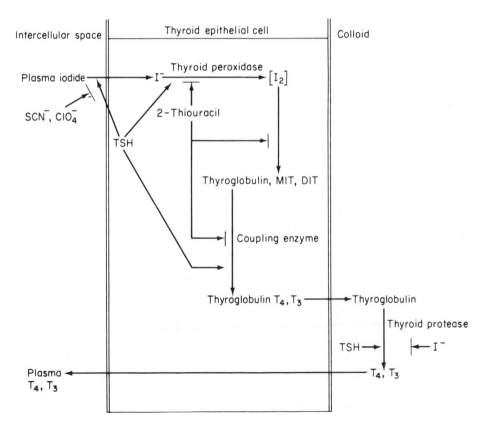

Figure 3.2 The biosynthesis of thyroid hormones in the thyroid gland, showing the effect of TSH and blocking agents, including the goitrogenic drugs. The movement of the various forms of iodine through the cell from the intercellular space to the colloid is represented. $[I_2]$ represents a postulated active form of iodine, as yet unidentified.

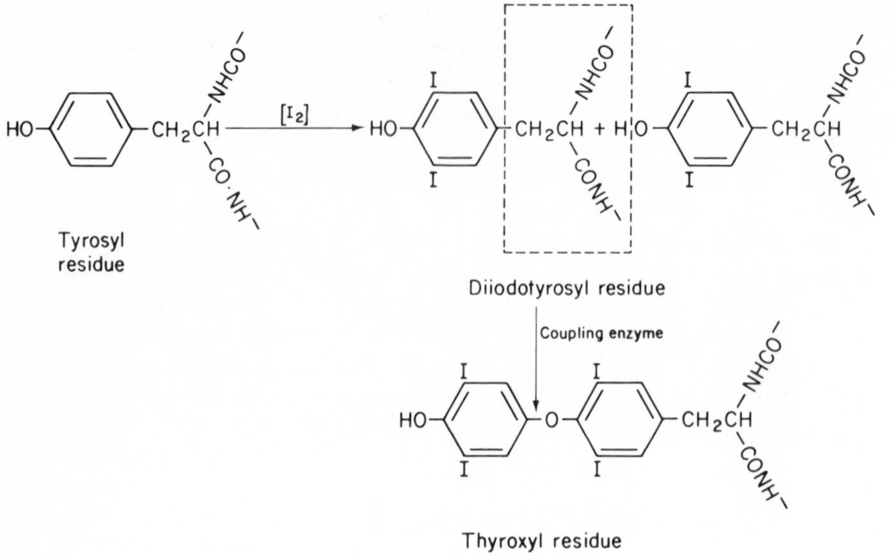

Figure 3.3 Proposed scheme for the formation of a thyroxyl residue from the iodination and condensation of two tyrosyl residues.

coupled, producing *N*-acetylthyroxyl-*N*-acetyllysine. In the thyroid gland, presumably two DIT residues combine to form T_4, whereas one MIT and one DIT
produce T_3.

The product of these reactions is thyroglobulin, a highly specialized protein
comprising the colloid of the follicle; it is a large glycoprotein, which has a molecular weight of 660,000 (19 S) and appears to be synthesized from four 6-S subunits
prior to iodination. Its relatively low isoelectric point of 4.6 is due to a high
proportion of aspartic and glutamic acid residues. After iodination, it typically
yields an average of twelve molecules of DIT plus MIT, two of T_4, one-third of T_3,
and traces of other thyronine derivatives (as shown in Table 3.1). Thyroglobulin is
completely digested prior to release of its amino acids into the bloodstream; thus
the organic iodide of the blood is predominantly T_4 and some T_3. In most mammals, the released hormone molecules are bound principally by three serum proteins: (1) T_4-binding globulin; (2) a prealbumin; and (3) albumin. Finally T_4 and
T_3 are dispersed, usually reaching a final concentration of 10^{-8} *M* or less in the
various tissues. As shown in Figure 3.1, TSH appears to exert a stimulating effect at
several points in T_4 biosynthesis; this includes the protease-directed release of the
iodinated amino acids into the blood.

3.2 STRUCTURE-ACTIVITY RELATIONSHIPS

Until the discovery of T_3 by Gross and Pitt-Rivers in 1952, T_4 was the most active
naturally occurring thyromimetic compound known. The fact that certain fractions

of thyroid gland preparations were more active than predicted from their T_4 analysis is now believed to be due to the presence of some T_3 and the better utilization of certain T_4-containing peptides. During the period from 1930 to 1940, Harington and his associates synthesized many of the conveniently accessible derivatives of T_4. They found that other halogens were active according to the series $I >$ $Br > Cl$, and that the diphenyl ether group was essential to activity. Activity was greatly enhanced by the 3,'5'-halogens, although it was later found that one halogen was better than two. The 1948 observations by E. Frieden and Winzler that certain side-chain analogs of T_4 had appreciable activity led to extensive studies of side-chain variants, many of which have activities comparable to T_3 and T_4 (Table 3.2). It was at first claimed that many of these side-chain derivatives, for example, T_3-propionate, were many times more active in the tadpole; however, this anomalous observation was later shown to be due to the unique immersion route used to test for activity in the tadpole. When tested by injection, the relative

TABLE 3.2 RELATIVE ACTIVITY OF THYROXINE AND
TRIIODOTHYRONINE ANALOGS

Analog *Thyronine[a] Derivatives*	O_2 *Consumption*	*TSH* *Suppression*	*Tadpole* *Metamorphosis*
L-Thyroxine (T_4)	1.00	1.00	1.00
D-Thyroxine	0.12	—	0.30
L-3,5,3'-triiodothyronine (T_3)	5.0	4.0	7.0
D-3,5,3'-triiodothyronine	—	—	3.0
DL-3,3',5'-triiodothyronine	<0.01	<0.01	0.03
L-3'-isopropyl-3,5-diiodothyronine	8.0	—	1.5
L-3'-isopropyl-3,5-dibromothyronine	7.0	—	2.0
DL-3,5,3,'-tribromothyronine	0.8	0.2	0.3
L-3,5-diiodothyronine (T_2)	<0.1	0.05	0.03
DL-3,3'-diiodothyronine	0.1	0.4	0.3
Side-chain analogs			
3,5,3',5'-tetraiodothyropropionic acid	0.5	0.4	3.0
3,5,3'-triiodothyropropionic acid[b]	0.2	0.5	7.0
3,5,3'	0.3	0.5	—
3,5,3'-triiodothyroacetic acid	0.2	0.5	7.0
3,5,3'-triiodothyroformic acid	<0.1	<0.1	0.5
3'-isopropyl1-3-5-diiodothyroacetic acid	0.4	—	5.0

[a] See Table 3.1 for the structure of thyronine.

[b] The structure of this compound is:

The remaining side-chain analogs vary only in having acetic acid or formic acid groups.

activities in the tadpole proved to be comparable to those observed in the rat, as shown in Table 3.2. A fascinating series of compounds with greater activity has recently been synthesized by Jorgenson *et al*. In particular, 3'-isopropyl-3,5-diiodothyronine was shown to be more active than T_3 and even the iodine-free analog, 3'-isopropyl-3,5-dibromo-L-thyronine is of comparable activity to T_3. Present data suggest that for the maximum thyromimetic activity, the thyroactive compound must conform to the structure schematically represented in Figure 3.4.

3.3 METABOLISM OF TRIIODOTHYRONINE AND THYROXINE

Our knowledge of the fate of T_3 and T_4 in the peripheral tissues is fragmentary. Thyroxine-glucuronide is apparently formed in the liver and excreted in the bile. The glucuronide can be hydrolyzed in the gut and reabsorbed, establishing an enterohepatic cycle (see Figure 3.1). There is evidence for many deiodinated products; iodide, 3,3',5'-triiodothyronine, 3,3'-diiodothyronine, 3'-monoiodothyronine, and thyronine. Efforts to establish that the deiodination of T_4 to T_3 is essential to hormone action have not been successful. Side-chain deamination, oxidation, and decarboxylation produce the acetic acid analog tetraiodothyroacetic acid (Tetrac.). Deiodination followed by ether splitting has been postulated, despite the obvious chemical problems associated with the latter reaction. The difficulty in studying

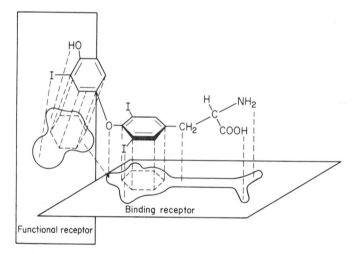

Figure 3.4   Representation of triiodothyronine interacting with a hypothetical thyroid hormone receptor. The binding receptor involves the 3,5-diiodotyrosyl residue while the functional moiety is represented by the 3'-Iodo and the 4'-hydroxyphenyloxy part of the molecule. [From E. C. Jorgensen, P. A. Lehman, C. Greenberg, and N. Zenker, "Thyroxine Analogues. VII, Antigastrogenic, Calorigenic, and Hypocholesteremic Activities of Some Oliphatic, Acyclic, and Aromatic Ethers of 3,5-Diiodotryosine in the Rat," *J. Biol. Chem.*, **237**, 3832 (1962).]

these reactions, which involve as complicated a substance as T_4, is compounded by the fact that T_4 appears to be uniformly distributed over many tissues and cells at concentrations of less than $10^{-7}\ M$.

3.4 EFFECTS OF THYROID HORMONES

The thyroid hormones regulate the metabolism of most of the adult bulk tissues—skeletal muscle, heart, liver, kidney—but do not normally affect the lungs, lymphatic system, gonads and accessory organs, nervous tissue, skin, smooth muscle, or thyroid gland (Table 3.3); in physiological doses, the thyroid hormones have a depressant effect on the pituitary. In these affected tissues, T_3 and T_4 show no fundamental qualitative differences in their action, although T_3 acts sooner than T_4 and its effects are of shorter duration. This has been explained on the basis that T_3

TABLE 3.3 SUMMARY OF OXYGEN CONSUMPTION CHANGES PRODUCED IN RAT TISSUE BY THYROIDECTOMY OR THYROXINE INJECTION[a,b]

Tissue	Percent Change Produced By	
	Thyroidectomy	Thyroxine
Liver	−20	+62
Diaphragm	−30	+73
Kidney	−15	+48
Salivary gland	−22	+34
Pancreas	−20	+51
Heart	−38	+132
Epidermis	−71	—[c]
Lung	+2	—
Brain	−2	+7
Spleen	−5	+3
Testis	+2	+13
Seminal vesicle	−3	0
Prostate	−1	+4
Ovary	−1	−2
Uterus	0	−3
Thymus	−9	+8
Lymph node	−2	+4
Gastric smooth muscle	+4	+3
Dermis	0	—[c]
Adenohypophysis	+49	−36

[a]Table from S. Barker, in R. V. H. Pitt-Rivers and W. R. Trotter (eds.), *The Thyroid Gland,* Butterworth Scientific Publications, London and Washington, 1964.

[b]These tests were made at least 1 mo. after thyroidectomy. Thyroxine was injected at doses of 1 to 2 mg/kg per day into thyroidectomized rats for 4 to 6 days and tissues were removed 1 day after the last injection.

[c]These tests were not made on thyroidectomized animals; neither epidermis nor dermis from intact animals injected with thyroxine showed a greater than normal oxygen uptake.

is bound less firmly to serum proteins (especially the thyroxine-binding globulin) and is thus more rapidly released to tissues than is T_4. The metabolic effects of T_4 and T_3 are therefore referred to interchangeably. Though the thyroid hormones have a distinct chemical structure, they induce numerous effects that may ultimately be initiated by a mechanism resembling that of other hormones. In common with growth hormone, insulin, and adrenal glucocorticoids, the thyroid hormones have a general stimulatory metabolic effect on numerous tissues in the vertebrates.

3.5 EFFECTS OF TRIIODOTHYRONINE AND THYROXINE IN THE GROWING MAMMAL

The essential role of the thyroid hormones in normal growth and development was dramatically emphasized when cretinism was associated with thyroid deficiency, resulting from iodine shortage or congenital thyroid insufficiency during infancy. The human cretin is a mental and physical dwarf with severely inhibited growth and maturation of the skeletal and nervous systems. The bones are infantile and abnormally calcified, and gonadal development is juvenile. The cretin manifests mental retardation, apparently due to the lack of both brain development and normal nerve growth. The basal metabolic rate is depressed by as much as 20 to 40 percent and the growth rate is reduced to less than 10 percent of normal. These multiple effects can be reversed by replacement therapy with T_3 or T_4, if administered sufficiently early in the growth period. Cretinism can be produced experimentally by surgical or chemical thyroidectomy of postnatal animals. While thyroid hormones are not required during early fetal life, they are involved in the later stages of fetal development.

3.6 INTERACTION WITH GROWTH HORMONE

There is a striking synergism between T_4 and GH. Pituitary function seems to be dependent on a minimal secretion of thyroid hormone—an amount insufficient to produce a detectable effect on the oxygen consumption of an animal. In the absence of thyroid hormone, GH can stimulate many of the aspects of normal growth, but adequate T_4 enhances the overall rate of growth. The thyroid hormone seems to be exclusively involved in the maturation of certain tissues—particularly brain, bone, and skin. In the hypophysectomized rat, both hormones are required for the growth rate to approach that of the normal rat. Also, administration of GH does not compensate for the absence of T_4 in the thyroidectomized rat; it is necessary to replace both endocrine secretions. The growth response to T_4 in thyroidectomized rats is due at least in part to a restoration of GH production and release by the pituitary.

Regarding the underlying mechanism involved, it is of interest that Widnell and Tata have recently found an independent stimulatory effect of both T_3 and GH on liver RNA (ribonucleic acid) polymerases. Their data emphasize the "permissive" effect of thyroid hormone on growth. The hormone permits normal growth and maturation; when absent, inadequate development occurs. However, it will not stimulate growth beyond the normal level, in contrast to GH. Although there is an upper limit in the growth response to thyroid hormone, excessive doses can produce an exaggerated effect on catabolic and oxidative metabolism with a large increase in oxygen consumption, a negative nitrogen balance, and a loss of weight. This is considered a thyrotoxic effect, distinct from the normal response.

3.7 EFFECT OF THE THYROID ON CALORIGENESIS

Historically, the action of thyroid hormone in vertebrate postdevelopmental stages has been associated with its ability to increase oxygen utilization and stimulate calorigenesis in many key tissues and organs; in adult homeotherms, its principal function has evolved toward thermogenesis. The rate of thyroid secretion is inversely related to the environmental temperature. Thyroidectomized animals are much more sensitive to the effects of cold; in human myxedema (thyroid deficiency in the adult), the heat-regulating mechanism is impaired. In fact, this calorigenic effect of thyroid hormones is a major contributor to the maintenance of the body temperature of homeotherms. The normal thyroid state of the animal provides the thermostatic setting for the metabolic rate. Other hormonal effects on metabolic rate are superimposed on this basal calorigenic level. However, in poikilothermic animals such as amphibia, the responses to thyroid hormone are not necessarily associated with calorigenesis, although an increase in oxygen consumption can be induced with large doses of T_3 or T_4. In these animals, the hormone induces and maintains the metamorphic changes leading to maturation.

Calorigenesis does not account for all the effects of thyroid hormones in restoring the hypothyroid adult to the normal (euthyroid) state. A more basic mechanism appears to be involved in the T_4 stimulation of RNA polymerase activity of liver nuclei from thyroidectomized rats. The rate of cytoplasmic protein synthesis is also reported to be increased by a thyroid-hormone-induced mitochondrial factor. Greater oxygen utilization may be viewed as the result, rather than the cause, of these metabolic events.

3.8 MECHANISM OF ACTION OF TRIIODOTHYRONINE AND THYROXINE

Few areas of endocrine research have generated as many frustrated efforts as the study of the mechanism of action of the thyroid hormones. The early emphasis on the role of thyroid hormones on metabolic rate led to an exhaustive study of the effects of T_3 and T_4 on oxidative metabolism and the intracellular energy-generating units, the mitochondria. There is no doubt that rates of oxidation and phosphorylation, along with their accompanying enzyme activities, are decreased in the thyroidectomized animal. These important reactions can be restored to normal by physiological doses of T_3 and T_4 (1 to 5 $\mu g/100$ g per day). In contrast, larger doses (> 50 μg/100 g per day) lead to exaggerated oxidative metabolism, uncoupling of phosphorylation from oxidation, and changes in mitochondrial structure that are evidenced by swelling. Effects of T_3 and T_4 at far greater than normal concentrations ($>> 10^{-7}$ M) have been observed on a large number of enzyme systems, particularly those of certain dehydrogenases and metalloenzymes, both in vivo and in vitro. However, since none of these effects has been directly related to the initiating mechanism of T_3 and T_4, it has been concluded that these are pharmacological effects arising from the intrinsically versatile chemical reactivity of these multifunctional molecules.

One of the earliest observed characteristics of thyroid-hormone action was the relatively prolonged lag period before metabolic or growth effects could be detected. It was apparent that certain key reactions must precede the later gross effects. With the growing understanding of the relationships between the nucleic acids (DNA and RNA) and protein biosynthesis, efforts to establish the site of thyroid and other hormone actions were concentrated on transcription and translation systems involving mRNA (messenger RNA) and *ribosomes*, the protein-synthesizing units of the cell (see page 151, Chapter 10). A familiar (though not infallible) test for dependence of biological phenomena on some aspect of protein biosynthesis is to determine whether they are sensitive to certain inhibitory agents, usually puromycin and actinomycin D. Tata, Sokoloff, and Weber were independently able to show that the calorigenic, growth promoting, and differentiating effects of thyroid hormones could be blocked by these agents.

Observations from these crucial experiments on the effects of thyroid hormones in both mammals and metamorphosing amphibia have led to a modern concept of thyroid-hormone action that accounts for the proper sequence of metabolic events. The temporal relationships of the thyroid-dependent reactions have been postulated (Figure 3.5). The rapid synthesis of nuclear RNA and the increased activity of RNA polymerase that is dependent on nuclear RNA both precede the incorporation of labeled amino acids into mitochondrial and microsomal proteins. Eventually, the increased synthesis and action of key enzymes result in an elevated metabolic rate and finally an increased amount of liver tissue. In the thyroidectomized animal, T_3 or T_4 is required for one or more of the rate-determining steps in protein biosynthesis; it may stimulate the biosynthesis of a broad spectrum of mRNA's, which in turn accelerate the biosynthesis of mitochondrial respiratory assemblies and microsomal enzymes. Although an accelerated RNA synthesis in the liver cells is an early event in the action of T_3, T_4, and GH, Tata has recently suggested that a coordinated sequence of changes in the protein-synthesizing machinery may take place before the biological effects of the hormones are expressed. The most prominent of these changes include increased production of ribosomes, increased amino acid incorporation into ribosomes, tighter ribosomal attachment to microsomal membranes, and proliferation of these membranes.

Another hypothesis, advanced by Sokoloff, Bronk, Hoch, and their co-workers, contends that the thyroid hormone effects on protein and RNA synthesis in liver cells initiate with the mitochondria and only later become reflected in changes in ribosomal and nuclear metabolism. Presumably these changes are followed by changes in cytoplasmic protein synthesis and structures.

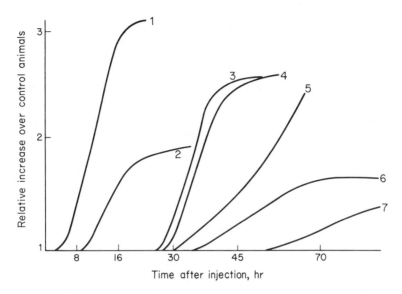

Figure 3.5   Proposed temporal relationship among the responses of some hepatic cellular activities, basal metabolic rate, and liver growth in thyroidectomized
rats following a single injection of 15-25 μg of triiodothyronine: (1)
synthesis of rapidly labelled nuclear RNA; (2) synthesis of DNA-dependent
RNA polymerase of the nucleus; (3) mitochondrial and microsomal incorporation of amino acids into protein; (4) synthesis of mitochondrial
cytochrome oxidase; (5) synthesis of microsomal NADPH-cytochrome c
reductase; (6) basal metabolic rate; (7) liver weight. [Data from J. R. Tata,
"The Formation and Distribution of Ribosomes during Hormone-induced
Growth and Development," *Biochem. J.,* **104**, 1 (1967).]

3.9   THE INDUCTION OF AMPHIBIAN METAMORPHOSIS

The induction of amphibian metamorphosis is one of the most dramatic effects of
thyroid hormone, illustrating its role in both differentiation and development.
Typical of amphibia, embryonic development results in a tadpole larval form that
differs greatly from the adult frog in both structure and habitat. This transition of
the tadpole to the frog during a discrete period of postembryonic change is known
as metamorphosis; this process is quite distinct from postmetamorphic growth and
maturation. Amphibian metamorphosis has become a model system for the study
of comparative biochemistry and cellular differentiation, especially since it illustrates a series of remarkable biochemical and structural adaptations. In 1912, F. G.
Gudernatsch showed that feeding thyroid glands to tadpoles initiated metamorphosis; this effect was eventually traced to T_4. Later, B. M. Allen demonstrated the
pituitary control over the secretion of thyroid hormone. More recently, W. Etkin
and A. Voitkevitch showed that pituitary activity is in turn dependent on signals
from the hypothalamus in the brain. If any of these tissues—thyroid, pituitary, or

hypothalamus—is destroyed, normal metamorphosis is arrested. Metamorphosis can be induced by T_3, T_4, or TSH. These hormones can even induce similar transformations in other amphibian species—for example, the Mexican axolotl—which does not metamorphose under normal conditions.

The extensive anatomical transformations during metamorphosis were described by biologists even before 1900. These changes reflect many millions of years of evolution. As shown in Figure 3.6, the frog tadpole resembles a fish, with a streamlined body and tail, gills, lidless eyes, thin skin, and a mouth suited to eating aquatic plants; within a period of several months it loses its fishlike characteristics and changes to a young frog, a versatile land animal with lungs, eyelids, thick skin, large limbs with powerful muscles, and a mouth and tongue adapted for capturing insects. Biochemical studies on the role of thyroid hormones in this process have been conducted only within the last 15 yr. Of the numerous biochemical systems known to be extensively modified during salientian metamorphosis, only several of the more dramatic molecular changes are summarized below:

Changes in blood proteins. An extensive adaptive change in homeostatic mechanisms that is mediated through the blood precedes the shift in environment. During metamorphosis, the amounts of serum albumin, copper protein, ceruloplasmin, and numerous other proteins greatly increase as a result of extensive changes in liver function. Tadpole hemoglobins are replaced by frog hemoglobins with a considerably lower oxygen-binding capacity, more suited to the new aerobic environment. Comparisons of these proteins reveal a number of significant differences in their chemistry. For example, in contrast to human fetal and adult hemoglobins, the tadpole and frog appear to have no hemoglobin polypeptide chains in common. Tadpole hemoglobins are unique in having no sulfhydryl groups, whereas frog hemoglobins have eight per molecule. Also, the site of reticulocyte formation shifts from the kidney (and possibly the liver) in the tadpole to the spleen in the frog.

Increase in tail hydrolases. During metamorphosis, disappearance of the tadpole tail is accompanied by large increases in concentrations of numerous hydrolytic enzymes, including cathepsins, deoxyribonuclease (DNase), ribonuclease (RNase), β-glucuronidase, phosphatases, and so forth. While other proteins disappear, these enzymes accumulate and produce tissue resorption.

The shift from ammonia to urea. A remarkable shift in the nitrogen-excretion pattern of the amphibian takes place during metamorphosis. As shown in Figure 3.7, over 90 percent of the tadple's nitrogen-excretion product is ammonia, characteristic of aquatic forms; this shifts to 90 percent urea after metamorphosis. Accompanying this shift from ammonotelism to ureotelism is a major increase in enzymes of the Krebs ornithine-urea cycle. One of the enzymes of this cycle, argininosuccinate synthetase, has been identified as the rate-limiting enzyme in the biosynthesis of arginine and, in turn, urea.

Basic initiating mechanism in the liver. Many of the changes mentioned above occur in the tadpole liver (such as those in the serum proteins and the urea-cycle enzymes), reflecting a major metabolic reorganization of this tissue during metamorphosis. In recent years, the liver has been utilized in the search for the basic mechanisms involved in the T_4 and T_3 effect on metamorphosis. As a result of the

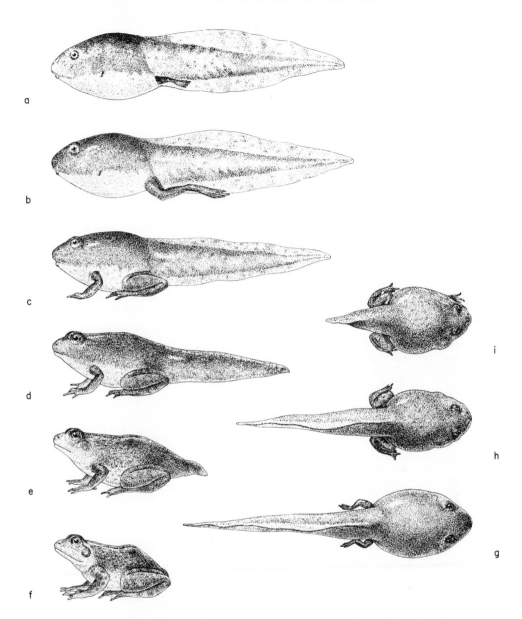

Figure 3.6 Metamorphosis transforms an aquatic larval form, the tadpole, into a ter-
restrial adult form, the frog. The later stages of spontaneous metamorphosis of the southern bullfrog, *Rana grylio,* are shown at left (a-f).
The animals were staged according to Taylor and Kollros (1946). Precocious metamorphosis, induced by treating a tadpole with thyroid hormone, is seen right : a Florida swamp frog tadpole, *Rana hecksheri* (g),
five days after injection with trace amounts of the hormones, thyroxine (h)
and faster acting triiodothyronine (i). (From "The Chemistry of Amphibian Metamorphosis," by Earl Frieden. Copyright © November 1963 by
Scientific American, Inc. All rights reserved.)

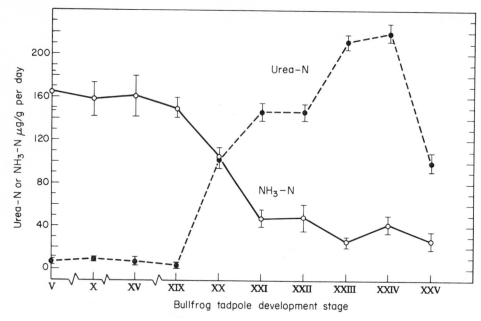

Figure 3.7   Urea-N and ammonia-N excretion at 25° C for different stages in the development of *Rana catesbeiana* tadpoles. Animals were staged according to Taylor and Kollros, *Anat. Rec.,* **94,** 7 (1946). See Figure 3.6 for examples of later stages. [Data from H. Ashley, P. Katti, and E. Frieden, "Urea Excretion in the Bullfrog Tadpole: Effect of Temperature, Metamorphosis, and Thyroid Hormones," *Dev. Biol.,* **17,** 293 (1968).]

studies of Cohen, Frieden, and Tata, and their associates, it has been shown that T_3 and T_4 can induce an increased RNA biosynthesis prior to many of the changes in protein metabolism cited above. Thus, in common with the mechanisms cited for the effects of thyroid hormones on liver tissue in the growing rat, RNA- and protein-biosynthetic mechanisms have been shown to be stimulated by thyroid hormones (Figure 3.4) in the metamorphosing amphibian.

REFERENCES

Frieden, E.: in W. Etkin and L. Gilbert (eds.); *Metamorphosis: A Problem in Developmental Biology,* Appleton-Century-Crofts, New York, 1968.

Physiological Control of Iodine Metabolism (Proceedings of the 1965 Gunma Symposium, Institute of Endocrinology, Maebashi, Japan), Tokyo Press Company, Ltd., Tokyo, 1966.

Pitt-Rivers, R. V. H., and J. R. Tata: *The Thyroid Hormones,* Pergamon Press, Oxford, England, 1959.

Pitt-Rivers, R. V. H., and W. R. Trotter: *The Thyroid Gland,* vols. 1 and 2, Butterworth Scientific Publications, London and Washington, 1964,

FOUR

INSULIN AND GLUCAGON

The formation of many digestive enzymes and the regulation of carbohydrate metabolism are both functions of the pancreas. The former role is performed by an exocrine secretion containing a number of enzymes; the latter by the endocrine secretion of two hormones that regulate the concentration of glucose in the blood.

The pancreas develops from the duodenum as two outgrowths that merge into one; it comes to lie transversely in the abdomen below the stomach with its head in the curve of the duodenum and its tail near the spleen. In many animals, the pancreas is a compact lobulated organ, but in the rat it is diffusely spread through the mesentery. The exocrine function of the pancreas is performed by epithelial cells grouped into hollow spheres (acini); these are drained by ducts that generally empty into the upper duodenum via the pancreaticoduodenal duct. The endocrine function of the pancreas is performed by the islets of Langerhans (described by Langerhans in 1869), which contain three different types of cells: (1) the a cells which produce the hyperglycemic factor, glucagon; (2) the β cells which produce insulin, the hypoglycemic factor; and (3) the d cells, the function of which is unknown. In dogs the relative incidence of the a, β, and d cells is 20, 75, and 5 percent respectively. However, the distribution of cell types in the islets is unequal, the islets in the tail of the pancreas being virtually devoid of a cells.

4.1 DIABETES MELLITUS

Polyuria (excessive urine formation) is a common symptom associated with disease. The term *diabetes* (Gr., *siphon*) is frequently used to denote the polyuric symptom When diabetes is associated with a urine of high specific gravity and high glucose content, the condition is called *diabetes mellitus*. (Generally the term "diabetes" refers to diabetes mellitus.) This metabolic disease, characterized by polyuria, polydipsia (excessive water consumption), and polyphagia (excessive food consumption), was known and described in ancient Greek medicine. Diabetic animals show a hyperglycemia and a consequent glycosuria because the reabsorptive capacity of the kidney is exceeded; the polyuria is due to the large amount of glucose lost in the urine, which causes an osmotic diuresis. Such animals also show a lipemia that is due to increased mobilization of fatty acids, a ketonuria that is due to a ketonemia caused by increased metabolism of fatty acids, and an azoturia that is due to increased gluconeogenesis.

Diabetes can be caused by ablation of the pancreas, as von Mering and Minkowsky showed in 1889, or by damage to the β cells of the islets of Langerhans by alloxan, a derivative of uric acid (Figure 4.1). A characteristic of diabetes mellitus is shown by a reduced glucose tolerance test. The normal blood glucose concentration in fasting animals is 80 mg/100 ml; one hour after drinking a glucose solution (500 mg/kg body weight), the glucose concentration rises to 150 mg/100 ml; in 3 to 4 hr it is again at basal level. Blood glucose concentration in the diabetic animal is above that in the control animal: the fasting concentration may be 150 to 200 mg/100 ml blood; it may rise to 400 to 500 mg/100 ml after the glucose meal and after 5 hr still be above the initial concentration.

Houssay showed that the severity of the diabetic syndrome in depancreatized dogs is alleviated by hypophysectomy. The reduced severity of the condition is due to decreased utilization of fatty acids and decreased breakdown of protein and

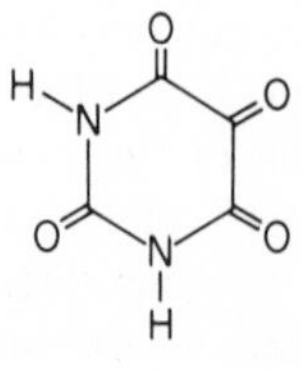

Figure 4.1

The structure of alloxan. This substance is highly toxic to the β cells of the pancreatic islets of Langerhans. The destruction of these cells results in diabetes mellitus, providing further evidence that the β cells are the source of insulin.

subsequent conversion to glucose (gluconeogenesis). A similar effect is obtained after adrenalectomy.

4.2 CHEMISTRY OF INSULIN

Almost 50 years have elapsed since Banting and Best demonstrated that extracts of the pancreas could cause hypoglycemia in diabetic dogs. Their success where others had failed was due to Banting's realization that the proteolytic enzymes of the pancreas destroyed the hormone involved. By ligating the pancreatic ducts of dogs, they destroyed the acinar tissue without damaging the islet tissue, which they then extracted. Abel crystallized insulin in 1926; 3 decades later, Sanger (1955) determined the complete amino acid sequence of bovine insulin (Figure 4.2). This was confirmed in 1964 through the synthesis of insulin by Katsoyannis *et al.*

Insulin derived from bovine pancreas has a molecular weight of 5,734 and is composed of two polypeptide chains designated A and B. The A chain has 21 amino acid residues, and the B chain has 30. The chains are connected to each other by disulfide bonds between cysteine residues at the A-7 and B-7 positions and at the A-20 and B-19 positions. The A chain also has a disulfide ring between cysteine residues at A-6 and A-11 (Figure 4.2). Structure-activity relationships indicate that the amino acid composition of this disulfide ring is not crucial to the activity of the parent molecule; in fact, it is one of the points of species variation (Table 4.1). The ring is composed of five amino acids, as is the disulfide ring of the neurohypophyseal hormones.

TABLE 4.1 SPECIES VARIATIONS OF THE A AND B
CHAINS OF INSULIN[a]

Species	A Chain (Disulfide Ring)	B Chain (C Terminal)
Ox	$\overset{6\ \ \ 7\ \ \ 8\ \ \ 9\ \ 10\ \ 11}{\text{-cys-cys-ala-ser-val-cys-}}$ $\underset{\text{S--S}}{\rule{0pt}{0pt}}$	30 -ala -ala
Sheep	-ala-gly-val-	-ala
Horse	-thr-gly-ile-	-ala
Pig, dog, whale (sperm)	-thr-ser-ile-	-ala
Rabbit	-thr-ser-ile-	-ser
Human	-thr-ser-ile-	-thr

[a] From F. G. Young, in U. S. von Euler and H. Heller (eds.), *Comparative Endocrinology*, vol. 1, p. 371, Academic Press, Inc., New York, 1963. Copyright © 1963 by Academic Press, Inc.

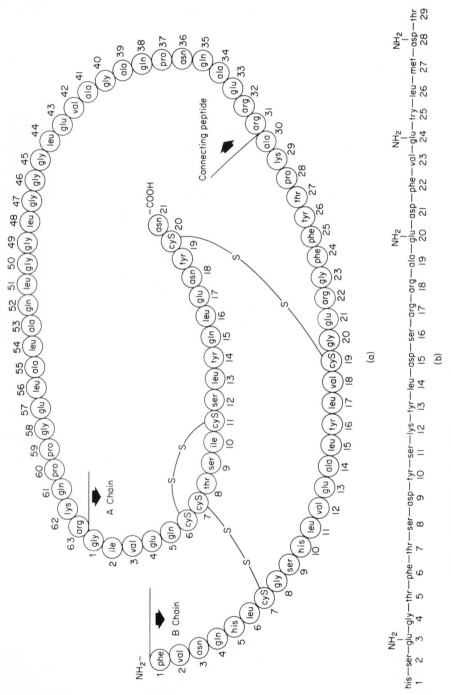

Figure 4.2 The amino acid sequence of procine pancreatic proinsulin (*a*) and glucagon (*b*). The proinsulin molecule contains within it the A and B chains of insulin. The molecular weight of porcine proinsulin is 9,082 [R. E. Chance, R. M. Ellis, and W. W. Bromer, "Porcine Proinsulin: Characterization and Amino Acid Sequence," *Science* **161**, 165 (1968). Copyright© 1968 by the American Association for the Advancement of Science.] Glucagon has a molecular weight of 3,485 [O. K. Behrens and W. W. Bromer, "*Glucagon*," *Vitamins Hormones*, **16**, 263 (1958).]

4.3 THE BIOSYNTHESIS OF INSULIN

The formation of insulin might proceed by (1) condensation of simultaneously synthesized A and B polypeptide chains, or (2) the cleavage of the insulin molecule from a macromolecule in which the polypeptide chains have been sequentially synthesized. Steiner has provided evidence that the latter hypothesis may be more correct. Slices of β-cell tumors of the human pancreas, known to cause hypoglycemia, were incubated with ^{3}H-phenylalanine or ^{3}H-leucine. Purification of the labeled protein and fractionation by gel filtration* caused separation of a protein with a large molecular weight (designated component b) from a smaller protein that had a mobility identical to that of porcine or bovine insulin. Limited tryptic digestion of component b yielded a radioactive peptide which, on gel filtration, had a mobility identical to that of porcine or bovine insulin. Sulfitolysis of the cleaved protein yielded labeled sulfonated A and B chains of insulin. Incubation of component b with large amounts of trypsin caused cleavage of the arginyl-glycine bond of the B chain and release of the heptapeptide B-23 to B-29. A similar approach with rat islet tissue demonstrated the presence of component b in this tissue also. During synthesis the appearance of component b precedes the appearance of insulin. Steiner has called this high-molecular-weight material proinsulin; its molecular weight was calculated as 9,082 on the basis of the complete amino acid sequence (Figure 4.2).

4.4 CHEMISTRY OF GLUCAGON

Murlin suggested in 1924 that the initial hyperglycemia seen after administration of insulin to normal dogs was due to a hyperglycemic contaminant, which he called glucagon. The insulin prepared by Abel caused no hyperglycemia, thereby supporting Murlin's idea. However, the commercial method of preparation in the United States resulted in a product that contained a hyperglycemic contaminant. Bouckaert and DeDuve showed in 1947 that insulin obtained from European sources lacked the hyperglycemic contaminant. In 1952, Staub used the residue from an insulin isolation to prepare a crystalline compound that caused hyperglycemia and glycogenolysis in liver tissues; in 1956, Bromer and Behrens determined the amino acid sequence of this molecule (Figure 4.2). Glucagon is a polypeptide, consisting of 29 amino acid residues, with a molecular weight of 3,485. It can be destroyed by many proteolytic enzymes, but may be freed of insulin contamination by treatment with alkali to which it is resistant.

*Gel filtration is a method for separating substances of different molecular size, and therefore weight, by molecular sieving. The substances used in this technique have cross linkings that on hydration in aqueous solutions give rise to smaller gel particles with well defined pores. The diameters of the pores vary with the cross linking. The size of the excluded molecule is therefore a function of the pore diameter.

4.5 REGULATION OF INSULIN SECRETION

A number of stimuli have been found to induce the pancreatic secretion of insulin under in vitro and in vivo conditions. The primary stimulus is blood sugar concentration. Hyperglycemia induces an increased insulin secretion and glucose is the most effective hexose in the sequence, glucose > mannose > fructose > galactose. Ingestion of food initiates a secretion of insulin. Food in the stomach and duodenum causes secretion of three gastrointestinal hormones: (1) gastrin, which increases gastric secretion of hydrochloric acid; (2) secretin, which stimulates the secretion of a watery pancreatic juice; and (3) pancreozymin, which stimulates secretion of a pancreatic juice rich in enzymes. The administration of any one of these to dogs causes an increased secretion of insulin that reaches its maximum rate within one minute. Glucagon, administered in doses of less than 100 ng, also induces secretion of insulin. However, the increase in serum insulin occurs concurrently with the increase in serum glucose (Table 4.2). Arginine and lysine, leucine, and phenylalanine increase secretion of insulin. Both epinephrine and norepinephrine inhibit the secretion of insulin in dogs and man even when glucose is administered simultaneously with the catecholamine; epinephrine is the more effective of the two. Insulin secretion is regulated by the interaction of hormones with the β cells and by the action of blood sugar as a negative-feedback stimulus (Figure 4.3). Together these regulatory mechanisms constitute an extremely sensitive control system, resulting in the homeostasis of glucose that Cannon visualized almost 50 years ago.

TABLE 4.2 EFFECTS OF GASTROINTESTINAL HORMONES ON GLUCOSE AND PANCREATIC SECRETIONS[a]

Hormone Dose	Arterial Glucose	Insulin Secretion	Glucagon Secretion
Glucagon, 1 μg	Prompt 50 mg/100 ml rise; peak at 6 min.	Prompt 250% rise; peak at 6 min.	
Secretin, 20–30 U (1–2 μg)	No effect	Vertical 290% rise; peak at 1 min.	None
Gastrin, 0.13–0.2 U (30–34 mg)	No effect	Vertical 390% rise; peak at 1 min.	None, or very slight
Pancreozymin-cholecystokinin, 100 U (17 μg)	Late rise; peak at 10 min.	Vertical 480% rise; peak at 1 min.	Prompt 80% rise; peak at 3 min.

[a]Data taken from R. H. Unger, H. Ketterer, J. Dupre, and A. M. Eisentraut, *J. Clin. Invest.*, **46**, 630–645 (1967).

4.6 REGULATION OF GLUCAGON SECRETION

Secretion of glucagon by the *a* cells of the pancreas is stimulated by hypoglycemia. Foa demonstrated by cross-circulation experiments between the pancreatic and femoral veins that induction of hypoglycemia in a donor dog caused the appearance of a phosphorylase-activating substance in the pancreatic vein that caused hyperglycemia in the recipient dog. While blood sugar concentration is the most potent regulator of glucagon secretion, pancreozymin is also effective (Figure 4.3). Although it causes secretion of both insulin and glucagon, pancreozymin is about six times more effective in inducing insulin secretion. Glucagon-immunoreactive material has been found in extracts of the gut; these extracts have shown glucagon-like biological activity. The source of intestinal glucagon is not known.

Unlike their role in response to stress (see Figure 1.1), the catecholamines are not involved in normal glucose homeostasis. Glucagon is a much more effective regulator of glucose release from the liver than is epinephrine. Sokol has emphasized

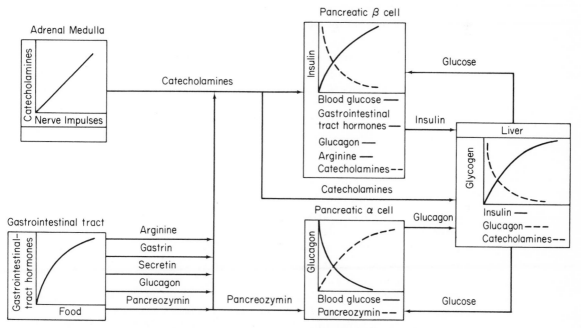

Figure 4.3 The regulation of blood sugar is mediated principally by insulin and glucagon in the liver. The action of insulin in muscle and adipose tissue as well as in other tissue is omitted. The liver is the only source of glucose in response to the action of glucagon and potentially almost all tissues, including liver, serve as sinks in response to the action of insulin. The catecholamines inhibit β-cell secretion of insulin but stimulate increased release of glucose by the liver. The increase in the concentrations of circulating gastrointestinal-tract hormones provide additional control on the regulation of β-cell secretion.

that while 10^{-6} M glucagon induces an increase in liver phosphorylase activity and glycogenolysis, 10^{-5} M ephinephrine is required for an equivalent effect.

4.7 EFFECT OF INSULIN ON CARBOHYDRATE METABOLISM

Insulin affects the metabolism of glucose, fatty acids, and amino acids. Its actions are so diverse that it could be considered a general metabolic hormone, modifying the utilization of nutrients in the same way that thyroid hormones in adult mammals modify the rate at which energy is released from these nutrients.

The formation of glucose-6-phosphate is of key importance in glucose metabolism: synthesis of glycogen (glycogenesis); degradation to pyruvate (glycolysis); and formation of pentoses via the pentose shunt. The pool of glucose-6-phosphate is maintained by entrance of glucose into the cell and phosphorylation to glucose-6-phosphate, and by conversion of glycerol and amino acids to glucose (gluconeogenesis). The enzymes capable of performing all of these reactions are found in the liver and perhaps in the kidney. Although the enzymes involved in glycolysis are also found in muscle and adipose tissue, these tissues can neither release glucose (because they lack glucose-6-phosphatase) nor form it (because they lack the transaminases necessary for gluconeogenesis; see Figure 4.4).

Levine and Goldstein (1949) demonstated that insulin caused an abrupt increase of cell permeability to galactose in eviscerated, nephrectomized dogs. They later showed that this effect of insulin on cell permeability to glucose and other monosaccharides was stereospecific for D-glucose structure in the first four carbons, that is, D-arabinose and D-xylose. Studies by other workers confirmed that the rate-limiting step for the movement of glucose into muscles is at the cell membrane in the absence of insulin; in its presence, glucokinase-activated phosphorylation becomes rate-limiting. Glucose enters liver cells freely and phosphorylation by glucokinase is the rate-limiting step in the formation of glucose-6-phosphate. Diabetes or starvation causes a reduction in glucokinase activity; recovery of activity occurs after administration of insulin or feeding, respectively.

The formation of glycogen from glucose-6-phosphate requires transformation to glucose-1-phosphate, condensation with uridine diphosphate to form uridine diphosphoglucose (UDPG) under the influence of UDPG pyrophosphorylase, and the introduction of D-glucose into the 1,4-configuration of glycogen by glycogen synthetase (Figure 4.4). Glycogen synthetase is rate-limiting and is affected by the presence of insulin; it can exist in two forms, a D form and an I form, referring to its dependence on or independence of glucose-6-phosphate. In the presence of insulin the I form predominates and glycogen formation occurs in the presence of low intracellular concentrations of glucose-6-phosphate. In the diabetic liver, glucose-6-phosphate formation is impaired; since the glycogen synthetase is in the D form, little glycogen can be formed.

The rate of glycolysis is determined by the phosphofructokinase and pyruvatekinase reactions, which are metabolically irreversible and rate-limiting. The pyruvatekinase reaction is regulated by insulin. Pyruvatekinase activity is reduced in

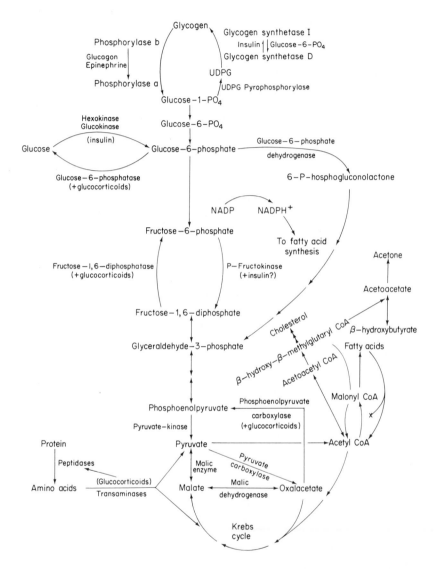

Figure 4.4 A diagramatic representation of the sites of control over the synthesis of glucose and glycogen. The interrelationships of the metabolisms of carbohydrates, fatty acids, and amino acids, the points at which they intersect, and the sites of hormonal activation of enzymes are shown. In no case is hormonal activation of enzymes understood. The reduced conversion of acetyl CoA to malonyl CoA is due to the inhibition exerted by higher fatty acyl CoA molecules on acetyl CoA carboxylase. Glucose-6-phosphate occupies a central position in this scheme since it provides a source of $NADPH^+$ for fat and steroid synthesis. It also provides smaller fragments for utilization of amino acid derivatives and for the complete metabolism of fatty acids. [Modified from B. R. Landau, "Adrenal Steroids and Carbohydrate Metabolism." *Vitamins and Hormones,* **23,** 1-59 (1965).]

diabetes, and restored by insulin; it varies directly with the carbohydrate content of the diet.

Fasting animals and diabetic rats show decreased activities of glucose-6-phosphate and 6-phosphogluconate dehydrogenases, and a decreased oxidation of glucose through the pentose shunt. A recovery of activity occurs about 12 hr after feeding or administration of insulin. This increase can be prevented by administration of actinomycin D or puromycin. However, since the rise in activity following administration of insulin can be prevented by imposing a fast on the animals, and since actinomycin D-treated rats are anorexic, it is not clear whether the insulin effect is due to increased availability of glucose-6-phosphate or induction of protein synthesis. The increase in fatty acid synthesis seen after insulin treatment may be due to the increased availability of NADPH* that results from the initial dehydrogenation of glucose-6-phosphate in the pentose shunt.

Gluconeogenesis is inhibited by insulin and stimulated by glucocorticoids (Figure 4.4). Diabetic animals have an accelerated rate of gluconeogenesis that can be reduced by adrenalectomy or insulin (Chapter 7, page 113). Gluconeogenesis is exaggerated in diabetic animals and is manifested by azoturia and muscle wasting; it can be relieved by insulin, hypophysectomy, or adrenalectomy. ACTH induces gluconeogenesis in hypophysectomized (but not in adrenalectomized) animals. The mechanism for this interaction is discussed in Chapter 7, page 113.

4.8   EFFECT OF INSULIN ON FAT METABOLISM

The fat stored in adipose tissue is derived from dietary fat or synthesized from carbohydrates; it is readily mobilized by numerous hormones, among which are ACTH, TSH, GH, glucagon, epinephrine, and norepinephrine. Mobilization of fat from adipose tissue involves hydrolysis of neutral fats by a lipase and the appearance in the blood of glycerol and free fatty acids complexed with plasma albumin. The fatty acids are readily metabolized by muscle cells, and in the fasting human the high concentration of free fatty acids in the plasma is associated with a respiratory quotient (RQ) of 0.77, elevated plasma GH concentration, and low plasma glucose and insulin concentrations.

In the fasting or diabetic animal, increased mobilization of fatty acids and lipemia result from formation of lipoproteins in the liver. The increased rate of fatty acid oxidation in the liver results in the accumulation of acetyl coenzyme A (CoA). Normally, the concentration of acetyl CoA is regulated by oxidation via the Krebs cycle and by synthesis of fatty acid or cholesterol (Figure 4.4). In starvation or diabetes, the pathways for oxidation and fatty acid synthesis are inhibited, the

---

*The following abbreviations are used: NAD, nicotinamide adenine dinucleotide; NADP, nicotinamide adenine dinucleotide phosphate; NADH, reduced NAD; NADPH, reduced NADP. In the older literature, NAD is often known as DPN (diphosphopyridine nucleotide), and NADP is known as TPN (triphosphopyridine nucleotide).

cholesterol pathway is open, and excess cholesterol synthesis ensues. β-Hydroxy-β-methylglutaryl CoA is found in the initial stage of steroid synthesis; it is the immediate precursor of mevalonic acid and the key compound in the formation of the ketone bodies. This coenzyme is formed by the condensation of acetoacetyl CoA; its cleavage produces acetoacetic acid and acetyl CoA. Acetoacetyl CoA is formed by the condensation of two molecules of acetyl CoA in the presence of thiolase. Acetoacetyl CoA and succinic acid in the presence of acetoacetyl-succinic CoA transferase give rise to more acetoacetic acid and succinyl CoA. In the diabetic liver, oxidation of acetoacetic acid is not readily accomplished; the excess diffuses into the blood. In the presence of β-hydroxybutyrate dehydrogenase and NADH, acetoacetic acid may be reduced, giving rise to β-hydroxybutyric acid. Decarboxylation of acetoacetic acid yields acetone. These three compounds—acetoacetic acid, β-hydroxybutyric acid, and acetone—are the familiar ketone bodies. Their appearance in the blood and urine causes ketonemia and ketonuria, respectively. The presence of acetone in the breath or urine leads to the diagnosis of ketosis. In addition to signs of deranged fat metabolism, ketone bodies cause a loss of Na^+ into the urine with consequent disturbance of acid-base balance of the blood, and a loss of water leading to dehydration.

4.9   EFFECT OF INSULIN ON PROTEIN METABOLISM

Insulin increases the rate of amino acid accumulation by muscle cells, probably in a manner similar to its effect on glucose uptake. This enhanced availability of amino acids may increase the rate of their incorporation into proteins. Insulin also affects protein synthesis directly by exerting an influence on the synthesis of macromolecules. In an in vitro system actinomycin D inhibits the biosynthetic action of insulin, but inhibition of increased amino acid transport occurs only after a long incubation period in actinomycin D.

Administration of insulin to rats causes an increased synthesis of RNA in the liver within 30 min and an increase in DNA between 24 and 36 hr. Growth of the liver is associated with the increase in DNA; over a 3-day period, the liver increases as much as 2.5 times in net weight. Liver RNA polymerase prepared from diabetic rats treated with insulin is increased in activity and may account for the rapid synthesis of RNA. After 36 hr, RNA synthesis in the liver changes in character and reflects the need for RNA in newly formed cells. The mechanism for activation of RNA polymerase is not known, nor is it clear that increased protein synthesis is due to activation of the sequence of events leading from transcription to translation. Wool has found that the 80 S ribosomes prepared from normal rat muscle are more active in polypeptide synthesis directed by polyuridylic acid than are similar ribosomes prepared from diabetic muscle. He suggested that decreased protein synthesis in ribosomes prepared from diabetic rat muscle is due to a defect in the 60 S subunit. The demonstration of the defect in the 60 S particle by this elegant experiment was based on the dissociation of the 80 S ribosomes into 40 S and 60 S subunits and subsequent hybridization of these subunits.

4.10 EFFECT OF GLUCAGON

Glucagon affects the kidney, causing an increased glomerular filtration rate and renal plasma flow, with a consequently increased excretion of ions. However, regulation of blood glucose is the primary role of glucagon. It can also, by virtue of its activation of adenylcyclase and consequent increase in the concentration of c-AMP cause lipolysis in adipose tissue. Glycogenolysis and hyperglycemia result from the action of glucagon and epinephrine on liver, whereas glycogenolysis and glycolysis result from the action of epinephrine on muscle. Both glucagon and epinephrine appear to activate the enzyme adenylcyclase, which converts ATP (adenosine triphosphate) to c-AMP (Figure 4.5). Unfortunately the inability to purify adenylcyclase, which appears to be membrane-bound, has interfered with an under-

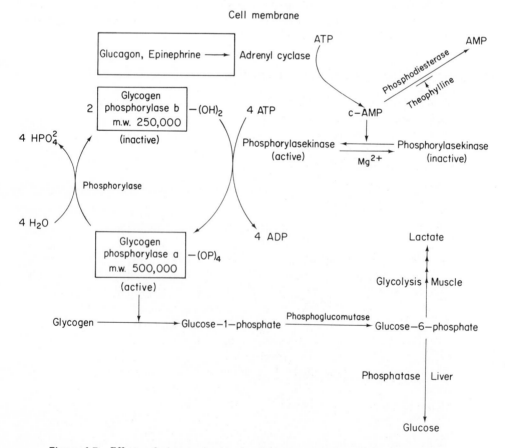

Figure 4.5 Effects of glucagon and epinephrine on c-AMP and the glycogenolytic enzymes of muscle and liver.

standing of the specific mechanism involved. Acting as a "second messenger," c-AMP regulates the conversion of an inactive form of phosphorylasekinase to an active form. Glycogen phosphorylase b is transformed to glycogen phosphorylase a, through the consumption of four molecules of ATP. Glycogen phosphorylase has been crystallized and its molecular changes are at least partially understood: there is an equilibrium between phosphorylase a and phosphorylase b; phosphorylasekinase is involved in the dimerization of two molecules of phosphorylase b, each having a molecular weight of 250,000, to one molecule of phosphorylase a having a molecular weight of 500,000. Concomitantly ATP phosphorylates four serine hydroxyl groups to serine phosphate (Figure 4.5). This appears to be a principal mechanism of intracellular control of glycogen phosphorylase, but other effects have been observed. For example, phosphorylase b can be made partially active in the presence of adenosine-5'-monophosphate. There is also a specific phosphorylase phosphatase which converts phosphorylase a to phosphorylase b independently of the phosphorylasekinase reaction. In muscle, glucose-6-phosphate derived from the degradation of glycogen is oxidized principally to lactate and further oxidation products. In the liver, which contains glucose-6-phosphatase, free glucose is formed. Diffusion of this glucose into the blood causes hyperglycemia.

4.11 SYNTHETIC HYPOGLYCEMIC AGENTS

Hypoglycemic agents other than insulin were first recognized in 1918 when guanidine was found to cause hypoglycemia; however, the toxicity of the agent precluded its clinical use. Although analogs of guanidine were prepared in 1926 and given clinical trials, their neurotoxicities were too great to permit application. By 1930, the hypoglycemic activity of sulfonamide compounds was recognized. In 1942, Janber and co-workers extensively examined the action of a thiodiazole-derivative of sulfonamide that caused extreme neurological disturbances in patients with typhoid fever; they noted that the disturbance was due to extreme hypoglycemia. The first compound with clinical usefulness was carbutamide, an antibacterial sulfonylurea compound introduced as a hypoglycemic agent by Franke and Fuchs in 1954. In stable diabetics requiring small maintenance doses of insulin, these synthetic drugs (Table 4.3) offer distinct advantages: they are effective when taken orally and are relatively free of toxic side effects.

The sulfonylureas exert two actions related to their effect as hypoglycemic agents: (1) they cause secretion of insulin when pancreatic-β-cell tissue is present; (2) they cause potentiation of administered insulin, as seen in the enhanced action of insulin in severely diabetic animals.

The guanidine derivatives cause hypoglycemia in the absence of the pancreas. Synthalin A causes transient hyperglycemia and then a marked hypoglycemia, due to a severe hepatotoxic effect. The biguanidine compound 1-phenethylbiguanide (DBI) does not cause a hypoglycemia in normal human subjects, but does in mildly diabetic subjects. Its action is not dependent on the presence of a functioning

TABLE 4.3 ORALLY ACTIVE HYPOGLYCEMIC AGENTS

Sulfonylureas:[a]

Carbutamide: N-(p-aminobenzenesulfonyl)-N'-(n-butyl)urea

$$H_2N-\underset{}{\bigcirc}-SO_2-NH-CO-NH-C_4H_9$$

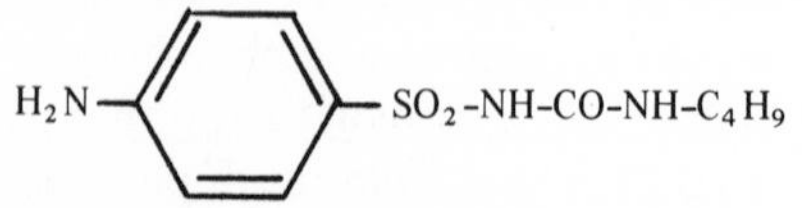

Tolbutamide: N-(p-toluenesulfonyl)-N'-(n-butyl)urea

$$H_3C-\underset{}{\bigcirc}-SO_2-NH-CO-NH-C_4H_9$$

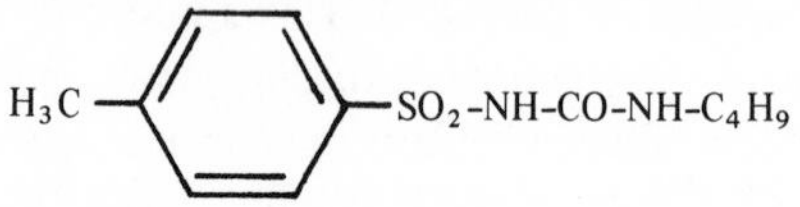

Chlorpropamide: N-(p-chlorobenzenesulfonyl)-N'(n-propyl)urea

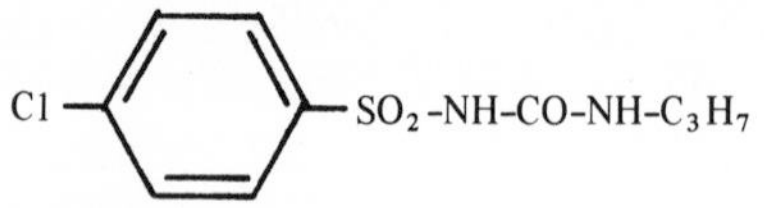

$$Cl-\underset{}{\bigcirc}-SO_2-NH-CO-NH-C_3H_7$$

Guanidine derivatives:

Methylguanidine:

$$CH_3-NH-\underset{\underset{NH}{\|}}{C}-NH_2$$

Synthalin A: decamethylenediguanidine dihydrochloride

$$H_2N-\underset{\underset{NH}{\|}}{C}-NH-(CH_2)_{10}-HN-\underset{\underset{NH}{\|}}{C}-NH_2 \bullet 2\,HCl$$

Synthalin B: dodecamethylenediguanidine dihydrochloride

$$H_2N-\underset{\underset{NH}{\|}}{C}-NH-(CH_2)_{12}-HN-\underset{\underset{NH}{\|}}{C}-NH_2 \bullet 2\,HCl$$

DBI: 1-phenethylbiguanidine

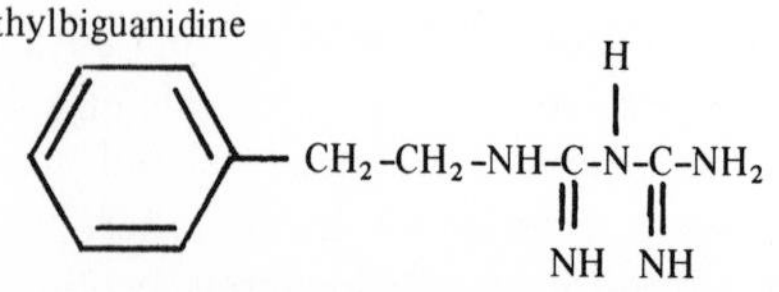

$$\underset{}{\bigcirc}-CH_2-CH_2-NH-\underset{\underset{NH}{\|}}{C}-\overset{\overset{H}{|}}{N}-\underset{\underset{NH}{\|}}{C}-NH_2$$

---

[a]The R_1-SO_2-NH-CO-R structure is essential for hypoglycemic effect: R_1 and R_2 determine duration and intensity of hypoglycemia.
The order of hypoglycemic potency is chlorpropamide $>$ tolbutamide $>$ carbutamide.

pancreas, nor does it potentiate the action of exogenous insulin in diabetic animals. No acceptable explanation for the action of DBI is present in the literature. One suggestion based on an in vitro study was that this drug, which depresses oxygen consumption, may promote the utilization of glucose by enhancement of anaerobic glycolysis.

REFERENCES

Duncan, L. J. P., and J. D. Baird: "Compounds Administered Orally in the Treatment of Diabetes Mellitus," *Pharmacol. Rev.,* 12, 31 (1960).

Goodman, L. S., and A. Gilman: *The Pharmacological Basis of Therapeutics,* 3rd ed., The Macmillan Company, New York, 1965.

Steiner, D. F.: "Insulin and the Regulation of Hepatic Biosynthetic Activity," *Vitamins and Hormones,* 24, 1 (1966).

Newshalme, E. A., and W. Geners: "Control of Glycolysis and Gluconeogenesis in Liver and Kidney Cortex," *Vitamins and Hormones,* 25, 1 (1967).

CHEMISTRY, BIOSYNTHESIS, AND STRUCTURAL RELATIONSHIPS OF THE STEROID HORMONES

FIVE

In Chapter 1, it was noted that hormones may be classified into three major chemical groups: (1) proteins and peptides; (2) steroids; and (3) a miscellaneous, less homogeneous group usually closely related to or derived from amino acids. The purpose of this chapter is to outline the chemistry, biosynthesis, and activity relationships of the steroid hormones.

Steroids are derivatives of an almost completely hydrogenated phenanthrene core [Figure 5.1 (I)] to which a cyclopentane group is attached, that is, a 1,2-cyclopentanoperhydrophenanthrene structure, a sterane (II). The most commonly occurring animal steroid (or sterol) is cholesterol (III), a complicated derivative of sterane with a hydroxyl group at C-3, a double bond between C-5 and C-6, a methyl group at C-10 and at C-13, and a methylated isoheptane side chain at C-17; its name is derived from the fact that it is a common constituent of human gallstones and is deposited in the bile (chole) duct. Cholesterol is in fact a major constituent of all normal tissues; an 80-kg man has about 240 g of cholesterol. It is a principal component of esterified lipids, the myelin sheath, and most cell membranes, in addition to being a metabolic precursor of most steroid hormones. By comparison,

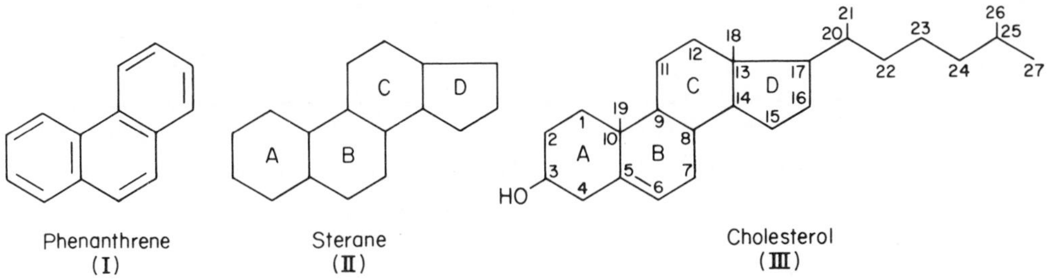

Figure 5.1   The structural basis of a steroid.

the common steroid hormones have fewer side-chain carbons but frequently more substituents than cholesterol. The principal categories of steroids to be discussed here are summarized in Table 5.1. Some of the commonly used nomenclature are summarized in Table 5.2.

TABLE 5.1   CHOLESTEROL AND THE STEROID HORMONES

Group	Parent Ring System	Principal Compound	Number of Carbon Atoms	Principal Source
Sterol	Cholestane	Cholesterol	27	All tissues and cells
Estrogen	Estrane	Estradiol	18	Ovary; follicles
Androgen	Androstane	Testosterone	19	Testis; interstitial cells
Progestogen	Pregnane	Progesterone	21	Ovary; corpus luteum
Mineralcorticoid	Pregnane	Aldosterone	21	Adrenal cortex; zona glomerulosa
Glucocorticoid	Pregnane	Cortisol	21	Adrenal cortex; zona fasicularis

5.1 CONFORMATION, STEREOCHEMISTRY, AND RING SYSTEMS

Since cholesterol is the parent sterol and accepted precursor of the five major classes of steroid hormones, its conformation, stereochemistry, and ring system as they reflect on the steroid hormones shall be discussed in detail. Cholesterol is composed of three fused cyclohexane rings (*A, B, C*) attached to a terminal cyclopentane ring (*D*) with a saturated, branched side chain at C-17. The conformation of cholesterol (IV) is pictured in Figure 5.2, with rings *B* and *C* locked rigidly in the chair conformation (V) by transfusion to rings *A* and *D*. Although ring *A* is theoretically free to change orientation, creating the boat arrangement (VI), the usual stability of the chair form is reinforced by the steric hindrance of the hydroxyl group at C-3 and the methyl group at C-10. As shown in IV, the ring fusions 5-10, 8-9, and 13-14 are *trans;* the bonds 9-10 and 8-14 are in the *trans* configuration. These structural restrictions give the steroids an outspread geometry (as in IV) not readily apparent from the convenient usual representation (as in III), and enhance its ability to serve as an integral part of cell structure, particularly in cell mem-

TABLE 5.2a COMMON NOMENCLATURE CONVENTIONS OF THE STEROIDS

Suffix or Prefix	Meaning	Example; Number
– ane	Saturated chain or ring system	**Androstane**
– ene	Unsaturation; one or more double bonds	Preg**nenolone** (XXXVIII)
– ol	Hydroxy group	Cholester**ol** (III)
– one	Keto group	Androster**one** (XLI)
hydroxy –	α – OH (below plane of ring)[a]	β – Estra**diol** (VIII)
α –, β –	β – OH (above plane of ring)[a]	
keto –	Ketone group	17 – **Keto**steroid (Fig. 5-13)
Δ^3 –	Double bond between C – 3 and C – 4	Δ^3 – Isopentenyl pyrophosphate (XXX)
nor –	One less carbon in side chain	19 – **Nor**testosterone (Figure 5-11)
allo –	Another form; rings *A* and *B* are *trans*	**Allo**pregnane
cis –	Two groups on same side of plane	———
trans –	Two groups on opposite sides of plane	———
oxy (oxo) –	One additional oxygen	19 – **Oxo**testosterone (Fig. 5-11)
deoxy –	One less oxygen	11 – **deoxy**corticosterone (XVII)
hydro (dihydro)–	Two additional hydrogens	**Hydro**cortisone (cortisol) (IX)
dehydro –	Two less hydrogens	7 – **Dehydro**cholesterol
epi –	Isomeric to named compound, usually in relation to stereochemistry at C – 3	**Epi**androsterone

[a] α substituents, which are below the plane of the ring, are indicated by a dashed line as - - -; β substituents, which are above the plane of the ring, are indicated by a solid line as ——.

TABLE 5.2b CORRECT CHEMICAL NAMES FOR SOME HORMONAL STEROIDS

Trivial Name	IUPAC/IUB[b] Complete Identification
Aldosterone	18, 11 – Hemiacetal of 11β,21 – dihydroxy – 20 – oxopregn – 4 – en – 18 – al
Androsterone	3α – Hydroxy – 5α – androstan – 17 – one
Cholesterol	5 – Cholesten – 3β – ol
Corticosterone	11β,21 – Dihydroxy – 4 – pregnene – 3,20 – dione
Cortisol	11β,17α,21, – Trihydroxy – 4 – pregnene – 3,20 – dione
Cortisone	17α,21 – Dihydroxy – 4 – pregnene – 3,11,20 – trione
Deoxycorticosterone	21 – Hydroxy – 4 – pregnene – 3,20 – dione (that is, the 11 – deoxy derivative of corticosterone)
Estradiol – 17β	1,3,5(10) – Estratriene – 3,17β – diol
Estrone	3 – Hydroxy – 1,3,5(10) – estratrien – 17 – one
Progesterone	4 – Pregnene – 3,20 – dione
Testosterone	17β – Hydroxy – 4 – androsten – 3 – one

[b] IUPAC, International Union of Pure and Applied Chemistry; IUB, International Union of Biochemistry.

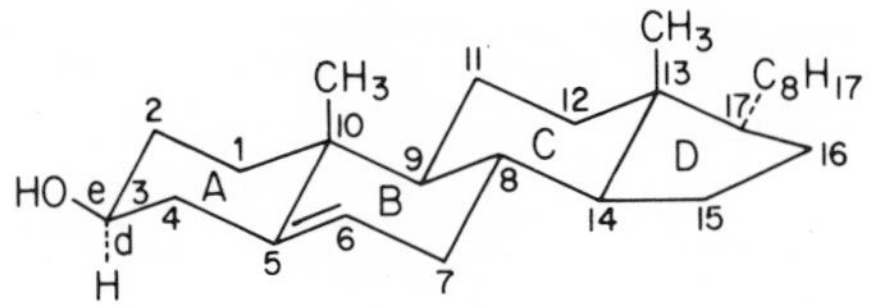

Cholesterol
(**IV**)

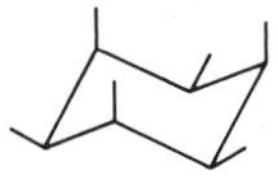

Chair   Boat
(**V**)   (**VI**)

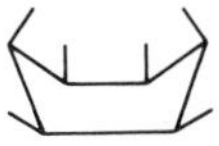

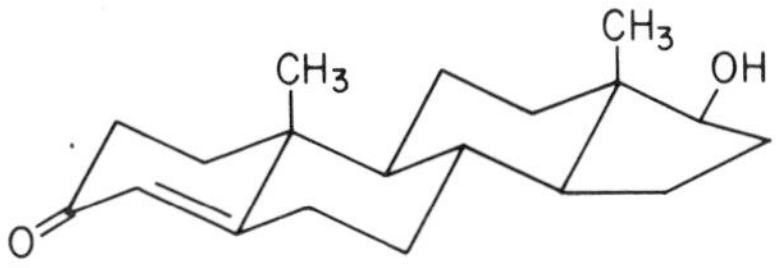

Testosterone (androgen series)   Estradiol (estrogen series)
(**VII**)   **VIII**

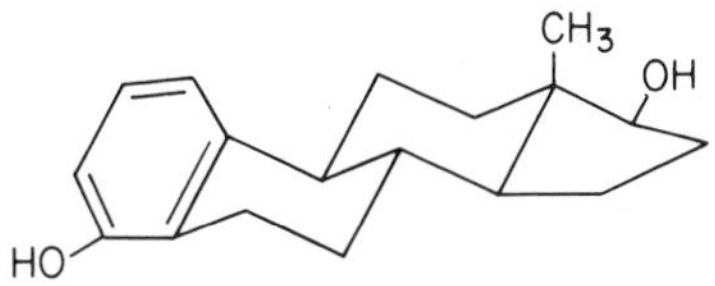

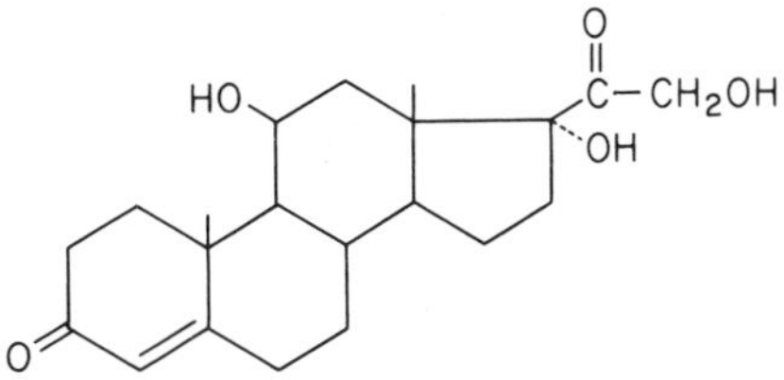

Cortisol (pregnane series)
(**IX**)

Figure 5.2   Conformation of selected steroids.

branes. The ring configurations of two other distinctive families of steroids are shown in VII and VIII.

It is now profitable to consider several of the other key features involved in the stereochemistry of the steroid hormones. The angular methyl groups at C-10 and C-13 are both found in all steroids except the estrogens (VIII), in which ring A is benzenoid and the C-13 group is retained. Since most of the steroid hormones have one or more hydroxyl groups attached to a saturated ring, two isomers are possible, often of widely different biological activity. In cholesterol, the 3-OH group is equatorial rather than axial, but 3β-OH groups are rarely found among the steroid hormones (except estrogens). The 17-OH group of both testosterone (VII) and estradiol (VIII) is β; the 17a-OH derivatives are known, but are biologically much less active. However, the most active naturally occurring glucocorticoid, cortisol

(IX), is a 17α-OH-corticosterone. In all natural steroids the chain attached to C-17 is also β.. Finally, a double bond at the 4-5 position is found in most of the active 3-ketosteroids, including testosterone, progesterone (X), and most of the adrenal steroids. Some other aspects of progesterone structure are also shown in Figure 5.3.

In the remaining parts of this chapter, the steroid hormones are considered from two major viewpoints: (1) the chemical features essential to their biological activity (with illustrative tables), and (2) their biosynthesis from typical precursors. Salient comments about their metabolism will also be included where significant.

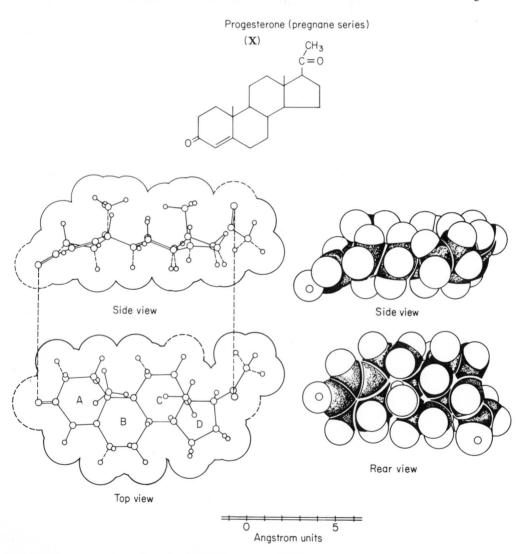

Figure 5.3   Stereochemical representations of progesterone. (From *Concepts in Biochemistry* by F. J. Reithel. Copyright © 1967 by McGraw-Hill, Inc. Used with permission of McGraw-Hill Book Company.)

5.2 THE ESTROGENS

The estrogens are steroids produced by the developing ovarian follicle. Their structure is unique in that ring A is benzenoid, requiring the elimination of the methyl
group at C-10. For maximum activity, the presence of alcohol groups at C-3 and
C-17β is essential. A 16α-OH, as in estriol (see Figure 5.12 on page 96) reduces
activity. The relative activity of several estrogens is shown in Table 5.3. The alcohol
at C-3 is phenolic and its weakly acidic character makes the estrogens soluble in
dilute base and responsive to certain other unique detecting reactions. These properties were instrumental in the isolation in 1929 of the first steroid hormone,
estrone [Figure 5.4 (XI)], from pregnant mares' urine by E. A. Doisy, of St. Louis
University School of Medicine, and A. Butenandt, of Gottingen University.
Estradiol-17β (VIII), the most active naturally occurring estrogen, was isolated in
1935 by Doisy *et al.,* although it had earlier been prepared synthetically by E.
Schwenk and F. Hildebrandt (1933). Subsequently, other estrogens—for example,
estriol and equilenin, with additional double bonds or hydroxyl groups—were isolated and identified.

During the early period of the growth of steroid hormone chemistry, prior to the
development of inexpensive synthetic methods, an attempt was made to devise
compounds of simpler chemical structure with high hormonal activity. The greatest

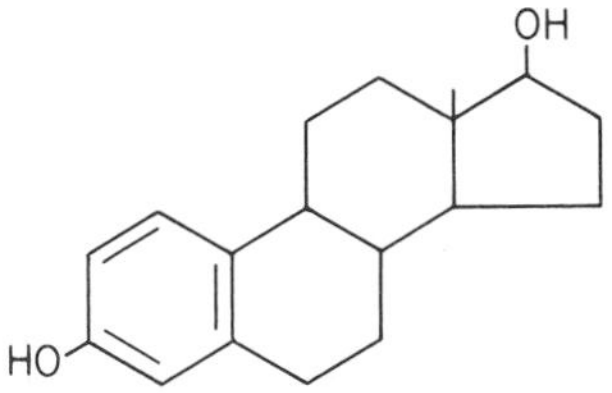

β–Estradiol
(VIII)
Estradiol–17–β

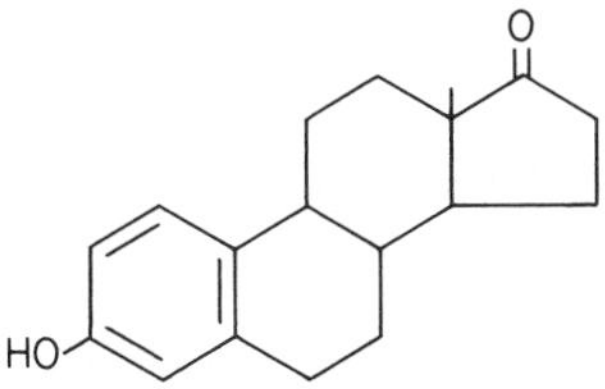

Estrone
(XI)

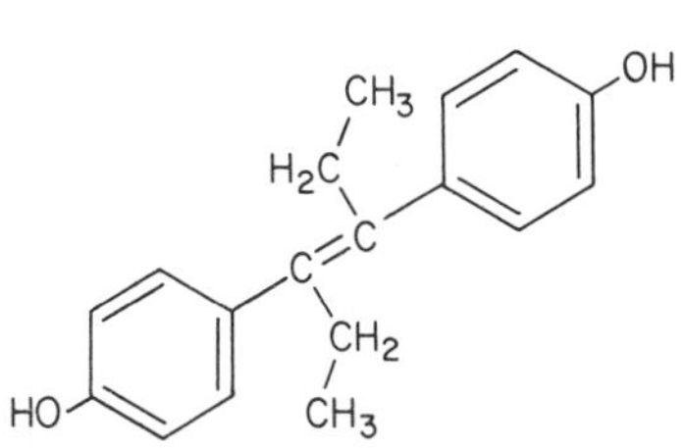

Dethylstilbestrol
(XII)

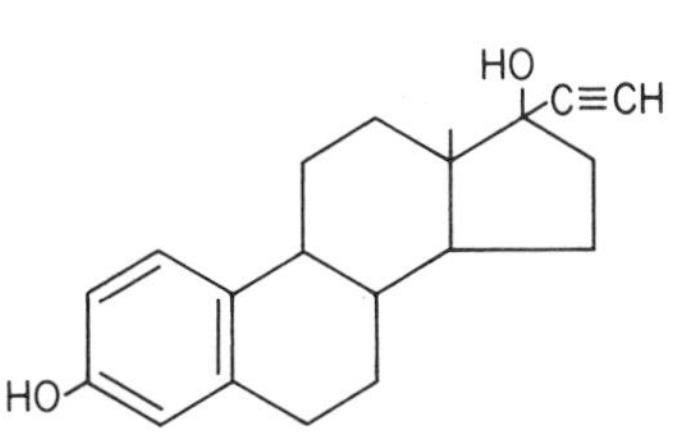

17–Ethinylestradiol
(XIII)

Figure 5.4   Natural and synthetic estrogens.

TABLE 5.3 COMPARATIVE BIOLOGICAL
                     ACTIVITY OF THE ESTROGENS

Compound	Mouse Test[a]	Rat Test
Estrone	1.0	1.0
β – Estradiol	10	10
α – Estradiol	0.08	0.1
Estriol	0.4	0.2
Stilbesterol	5	5

[a]The most sensitive mouse and rat test is based on the minimum dose necessary to produce nucleated epithelial or cornified cells in the vaginal smears of the ovariectomized animal. An effective subcutaneous dose of β-estradiol for vaginal response in mice is $0.02 \mu g$.

success in this area was achieved by Dodds and co-workers in 1933 when it was found that the compound diethylstilbesterol (XII) had unusually high estrogenic activity. This is a classical example of *isosterism*, a phenomenon in which a compound of apparently different chemical characteristics from the naturally occurring essential metabolite (for example, a vitamin, amino acid, or hormone) fits the physiological receptor system so as to substitute for the metabolite in every way. These synthetic estrogens have the advantage of exhibiting strong estrogenic activity when given orally. In contrast, estradiol-17β and estrone are so much less active by the oral route that a special group of orally active compounds have been designed, for example, ethinyl estradiol (XIII).

5.3 THE ANDROGENS

The androgens, of which testosterone (VII) is the most prominent example, are produced principally by the interstitial cells of the testes. As indicated in Figure 5.2, these are among the simplest steroids, having methyl groups at C-10 and C-13, a 4-5 double bond, a keto group at C-3, and a hydroxyl group at C-17. A closely related derivative, androsterone, can be made by direct oxidation of cholesterol. The story of the isolation and identification of these hormones from testicular extracts by Pezard (1911), Koch (1927), Butenandt (1931), and David *et al.* (1953) spans over 25 yr of intense effort in the field. All the other naturally occurring androgens have less activity than testosterone, including androsterone (see Figure 5.14 on page 98); however, a number of synthetic derivatives (Table 5.4) have been produced that have comparable androgenic activity and even greater myogenic activity (positive effect on nitrogen metabolism). The one exception to this is the 5-dihydro derivative of 5 α-androstone 32,17β diol, which has been recently identified as an intracellular metabolite of testosterone. Several of these compounds, such as 17-methyltestosterone, have the additional advantage of being more active than testosterone when administered orally. Certain simple testosterone esters, particularly testosterone benzoate, also have greater androgenic activity, probably because of protection of the 17-OH group or better absorption from the gut.

TABLE 5.4 COMPARATIVE BIOLOGICAL ACTIVITY OF
THE ANDROGENS

Androgen	*Dosage in Capon Comb Test,* *IU/mg*[a]
Testosterone	67
Androsterone	10
Dehydroisoandrosterone	4
Adrostenedione	10
17 – Methyltestosterone	83
17 – Ethynyltestosterone	110

[a]One IU of androgen is the amount that stimulates capon comb growth equivalent to that produced by 100μg of crystalline androsterone. In a typical test, single-comb cockerels, 48 to 72 hr. old, are injected with androgen on the lateral surface of the comb. Combs are removed and weighed on the eighth day.

5.4 THE PROGESTOGENS

The pregnane series, of which the principal representative is progesterone, is a slightly more complicated group of steroids. It should be emphasized that the C_{21} skeleton of the pregnane series is characteristic of not only the steroids with progesterone activity but also the major two groups of adrenosteroids: (1) the mineralcorticoids, and (2) the glucocorticoids. Progesterone is thus among the simplest biologically active C_{21} steroids, with keto groups at C-3 and C-20 and a 4-5 double bond. Because of the keen interest in orally active progestogens as contraceptive agents, a significant new group of highly active synthetic compounds has been identified (Figure 5.5); it includes chlormadinone acetate (6-chloro-17-hydroxpregna-4, 6-dien-3,20-dione acetate), which is over 2000 times as active as progesterone, and norethindrone acetate (17-hydroxy-17α-ethynylestr-4-en-3-one acetate), which is about 1000 times as active. These are either chemically modified progesterone or 17α-ethynyl derivatives of 19-norandrogens (the latter compounds are closely related to testosterone but lack the angular methyl group at C-19).

Because of their ability to delay ovulation, steroids of essentially progesterone-like character have served as the basis for the development of orally active contraceptive agents. A combination of an estrogen and a progestin is maximally active in preventing follicle maturation and ovulation, presumably because it inhibits pituitary gonadotrophin secretion. One of the earliest used formulas was a mixture of a predominant amount of norethynodrel (XIV), a compound with progesterone-like activity, with a small amount of mestranol (XV)—a synthetic estrogen—and another combination was norethindrone (XVI) with mestranol. When used daily from the fifth to the twenty-fifth day of each menstrual cycle, these compounds prevent conception. Recently, a once-a-month contraceptive pill has been developed; it consists of a combination of a long-acting, orally active estrogen—the 3-cyclopentyl ether of ethinyl estradiol—and 6,7 α-dimethyl-6-dehydroprogesterone.

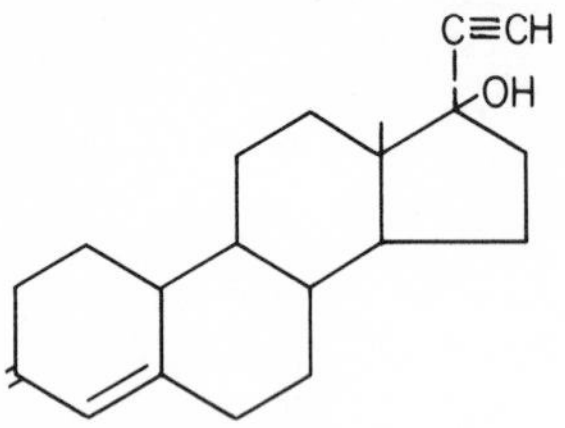

Norethindrone (norlutin)
(XVI)

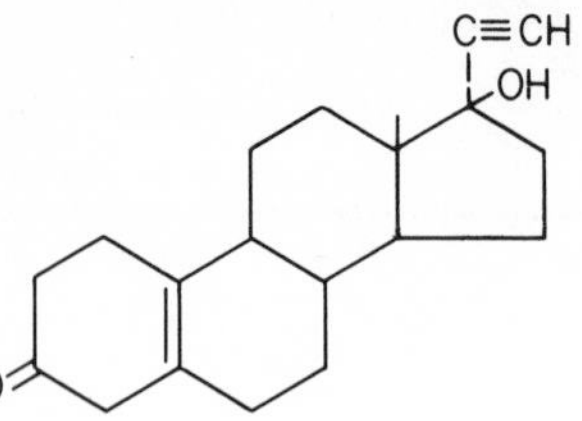

Norethynodrel
(XIV)

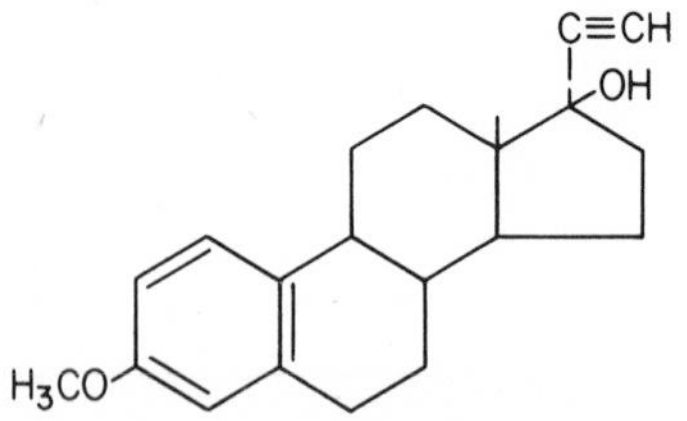

Mestranol
(XV)

Figure 5.5 Orally active contraceptive agents.

5.5 THE ADRENAL STEROIDS

The final group of steroid hormones prominent in mammalian systems is the adrenal steroids (Figure 5.6). These are basically progesterone derivatives with additional hydroxyl or oxy substitutions at C-11, C-17, C-19, and C-21. The adrenal steroids are commonly referred to as mineralcorticoids and glucocorticoids, to identify their two distinct major types of biochemical activity. However, most of the more than three dozen steroids isolated from the adrenal cortex have both kinds of activity, and a sharp delineation of precise structure-activity relationships cannot be made. Nevertheless, it will be useful to consider a few generalizations on this subject derived from the summary of data presented in Table 5.5 on the relative activities of natural and synthetic adrenal steroids.

The least complicated naturally occurring steroid having significant biological activity is 11-deoxycorticosterone (21-hydroxyprogesterone; XVII). It was once believed that this was the key mineralcorticoid since it maintains Na^+ levels essential to life in the adrenalectomized animal. But in 1953, mainly through the efforts of S. A. Simpson and J. F. Tait of Middlesex Hospital Medical School, London, aldosterone (XX), a complex steroid having by far the greatest mineralcorticoid

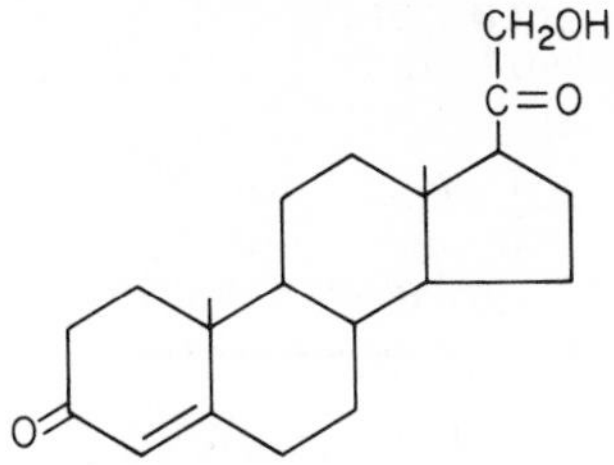

11-Deoxycorticosterone
(XVII)

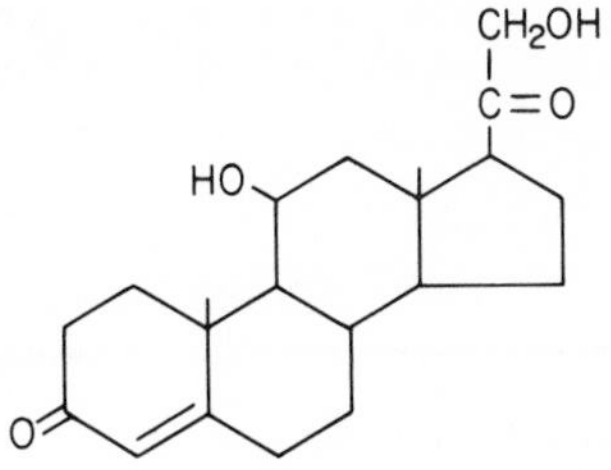

Corticosterone
(XVIII)

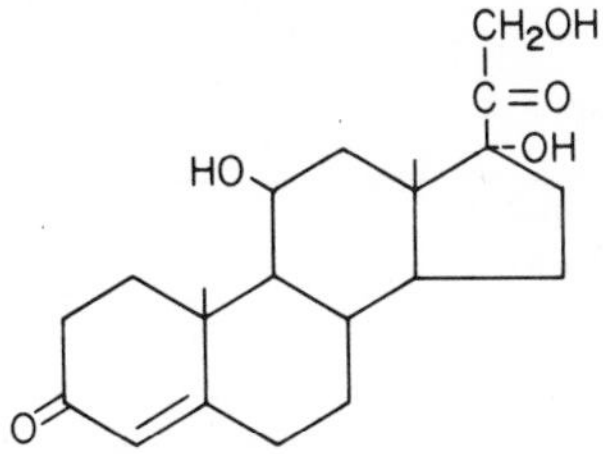

Cortisol (Hydrocortisone)
(IX)

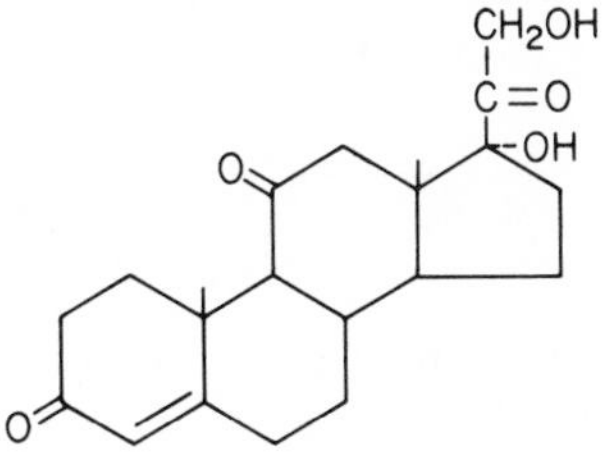

Cortisone
(XIX)

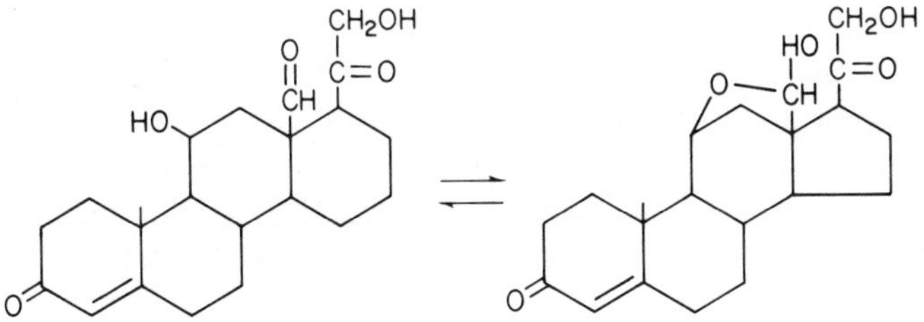

Aldosterone
(XX)

Aldosterone
(XX)

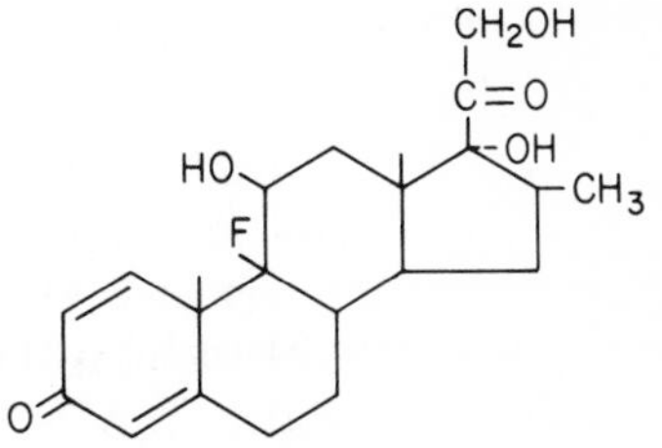

16α-methyl-9α-fluors-Δ[1]-cortisol
(Synthetic)
(XXI)

Figure 5.6 Structure of representative adrenal steroids.

activity, was isolated in crystalline form. Aldosterone has a unique aldehyde substitution at C-19, leading to a potential new C_5 ring with the C-11 oxygen. Although it was first believed that this structure was a requirement for maximum Na^+ retention, closely related steroids have been synthesized with the 2-methyl or 9-fluoro substituents, which confer similar mineralcorticoid activity (for example, XXI).

Glucocorticoid activity appears to be totally dependent on the 11-hydroxyl or 11-oxy group and enhanced by the 17-hydroxyl substitution and is best exemplified by cortisol [Figure 5.6 (IX)], the most prevalent natural glucocorticoid.

TABLE 5.5 BIOLOGICAL ACTIVITIES OF REPRESENTATIVE ADRENOCORTICAL
AND SYNTHETIC STEROIDS IN ADRENALECTOMIZED RATS

Steroid	Life Maintenance[a]	Sodium Retention[b]	Liver Glycogen Deposition[c]	Anti-inflam-matory Activity[d]
Cortisol	1.0	1.0	1.0	1.0
Cortisone	1.0	0.7	0.7	<0.6
11 – Deoxycorticosterone	4.0	10	<0.01	<0.01
Corticosterone	0.75	1.6	0.30	0.3
Aldosterone	80	300	0.30	0.
Δ^1 – Cortisol (prednisolone)	2.0	1.0	4.0	3.0
2α – methyl – 9α – fluorocortisol	–	1000	10	10
16α – methyl – 9α – fluoro – Δ^1 – cortisol	–	0.1 (minimal)	17	28

[a] Based on the survival of adrenalectomized rats maintained on limited-salt and water diet; a life maintenance dose of cortisol is 2 mg/100g per day.

[b] Based on the Na^+ and K^+ excretion of the adrenalectomized rat after controlled salt and water intake.

[c] Based on the amount of liver glycogen 1 hr. after a series of glucocorticoid injections in adrenalectomized, fasting mice or rats. An effective dose of cortisol is $100\mu g/100g$.

[d] Based on the reduction of the size of a granuloma (fibrotic deposit) produced by an irritant (small cotton ball) in the wound of an adrenalectomized rat after treatment with adrenal steroids.

Synthetic corticoids show a remarkable intensification of both glycogen deposition and antiinflammatory activity. The latter property is the most useful clinically. Compounds with strong glucocorticoid activity and minimal Na^+ retention activity have been synthesized, culminating in the compound $16a$-methyl-$19a$-fluoro-Δ^1-cortisol (XXI).

Only a small number of the 43 steroids identified in adrenal gland extracts have been considered here. E. C. Kendall and T. Reichstein shared the 1952 Nobel Prize in medicine (with P. Hench) for their major contributions to the isolation and identification of these important hormones. In addition to cortisol (IX), cortisone (XIX), corticosterone (XVIII), deoxycorticosterone (XVII), and aldosterone (XX), several other compounds appear in significant quantity, including 11-dehydrocorticosterone, and $17a$-hydroxydeoxycorticosterone. While virtually all these steroids have some degree of glucocorticoid and mineralcorticoid activity, other steroids with mild androgenic activity are also found, particularly adrenosterone, 4-androstene-3,17-dione, and androstene-3β,11β-diol-17-one. The production of these and other compounds with androgenic activity becomes exaggerated in certain adrenal tumors; women with such tumors develop secondary male characteristics sometimes leading to hirsutism and growth of beards. To further emphasize the overlap in steroid biosynthesis by the adrenals, it should be added that estrone, progesterone, and $17a$-hydroxyprogesterone also have been identified among the many adrenal steroids.

5.6   ECDYSONE—THE INSECT MOULTING HORMONE

Though there is a dearth of chemical information about the biosynthesis of ecdysone, this insect hormone was first obtained in crystalline form by Butenandt and
Karlson in 1958, and has now been identified as a steroid [Figure 5.7 (XXII)] with
a cholesterol-like side chain, five hydroxyl groups, one keto group, and a 7-8 double
bond. A variation of this structure, crustecdysone, has already been found in cer-

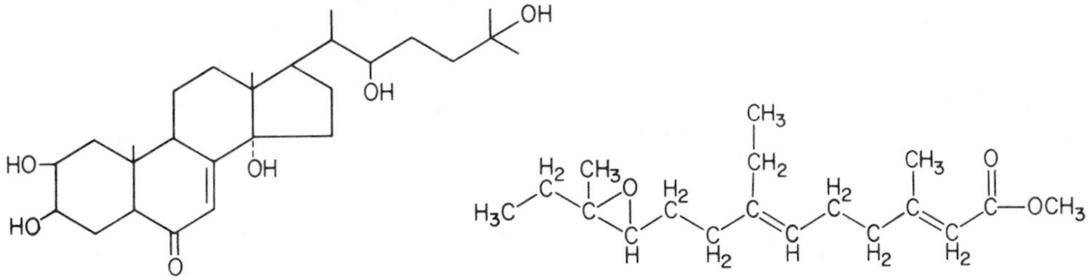

Ecdysone
XXII

Juvenile hormone
XXIII

Figure 5.7   Two important insect hormones.

tain crustacea. Insects cannot synthesize sterols from convenient carbohydrate or
lipid precursors; they need preformed cholesterol or sitosterol [particularly cecro-
pia (a silk-spinning moth)] as ecdysone precursors. None of the other insect or
plant hormones is currently believed to be a steroid, although the juvenile hormones comprise a family of compounds with modified linear isoprenoid units
(XXIII).

5.7   BIOSYNTHESIS OF THE STEROIDS

This discussion of steroid biosynthesis was reserved until now so that we could
first consider the steroids in detail and emphasize the close structural relationships
between the five major types of steroid hormones. In fact, the steroids appear to
have enough common precursors and metabolic pathways so that we may consider
their biosynthesis and metabolism together. In vertebrates, the principal direct
precursor of the steroids is cholesterol, the structure of which has been described
earlier. The objective here is to emphasize the paths from cholesterol to the various
steroid hormones; however, we should note that our present-day knowledge of the
biosynthesis of cholesterol represents an outstanding achievement (summarized below in Figure 5.9). The pioneering work, mainly of R. Schoenheimer, D. Ritten-
berg, and K. Bloch (Nobel prize winner in medicine and physiology, 1964),
established that most tissues can make cholesterol from acetate and other simple
precursors; the gonads, adrenals, liver, and skin are most active. Experiments with

labeled acetate have revealed that of the 27 carbons of cholesterol, 15 arise from the methyl and 12 from the carboxyl groups of acetate, as shown in Figure 5.8.

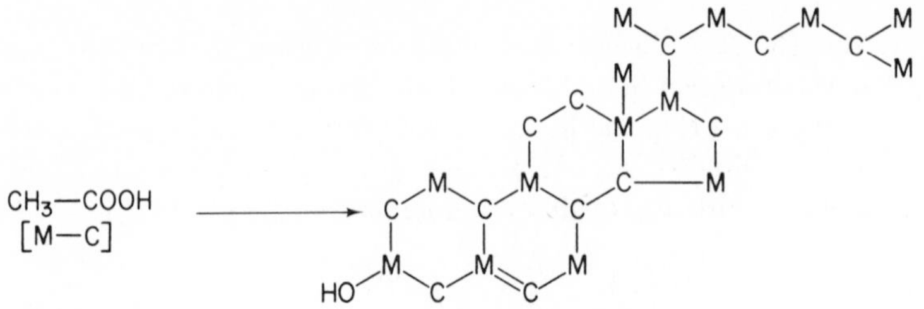

Figure 5.8   Source of the carbon atoms of cholesterol. The different carbon atoms are shown to be derived from either the methyl (M) carbon atom or the carboxyl (C) group of acetate.

The early synthetic steps involve metabolites activated as CoASH derivatives. Several of these intermediates correspond to those involved in the cytoplasmic synthesis of fatty acids. After mevalonic acid (XXVII) formation, cholesterol biosynthesis switches from C_2 addition to the condensation of six phosphorylated isoprenoid C_5 units using the active intermediate, isophentenyl pyrophosphate (XXX). Mevalonic acid also serves as a precursor for the carotenoids, coenzyme Qs, and the rubber hydrocarbons. Several alternative pathways are available for the formation of these active C_5 units. The overall reaction for cholesterol formation is:

$$18 \text{ Acetate} + 7 \text{ NADPH} + 6 \text{ ATP} \xrightarrow[\text{H}^+]{\text{CoASH}} \text{Cholesterol} + 6 \text{ CO}_2 + 7 \text{ NADP} + 6 \text{ ADP} + 6 \text{ P}_i$$

5.8   CONVERSION OF ACETATE TO CHOLESTEROL

The remarkable biosynthesis of cholesterol (Figure 5.9) is initiated by a series of reductive addition reactions, originating with the active C_2 unit, acetyl CoA (XXIV). Three molecules of acetylCoA condense to form β-*hydroxy*-β-methylglutaryl CoA (XXVI), which is reduced by NADPH to mevalonic acid (XXVII). Mevalonic acid is sequentially phosphorylated by ATP and then decarboxylated to 3-isopentenyl pyrophosphate (XXX), the major biological isoprene-interconverting unit. Isopentenyl pyrophosphate (XXX) is a nucleophile because of its terminal, doubly-bound methylene carbon. It is in equilibrium with a protonated form, dimethylallyl pyrophosphate (XXXa), which is electrophilic by virtue of its double bond and esterification with a strong acid. These two C_5 units are ideally suited for a head-to-tail condensation leading to a C_{10} intermediate, geranyl pyrophosphate (XXXI), and successively to a C_{15} compound, farnesyl pyrophosphate (XXXII). In these transformations a reactive allyl pyrophosphate is always regenerated, permitting continuous condensation and lengthening of chains,

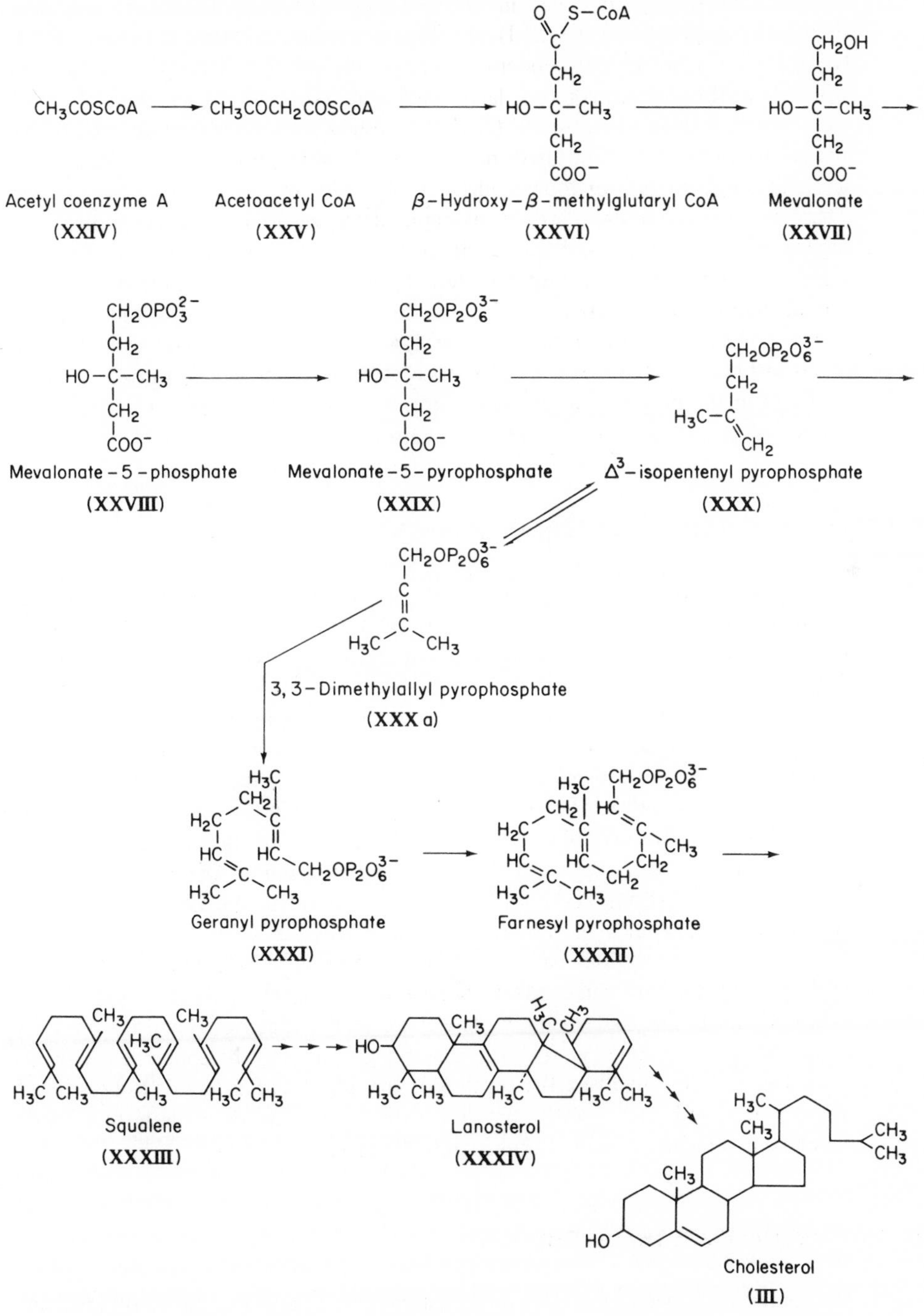

Figure 5.9 Biosynthesis of cholesterol from acetate, showing some key intermediates.

a mechanism widely employed in the formation of biological isoprene polymers. Farnesyl pyrophosphate (XXXII), an acyclic terpene, is then reductively (with NADPH) and symmetrically condensed to yield squalene (XXXIII), a C_{30} compound, which is a direct precursor to a large number of polycyclic triterpenes. The next step, from squalene to lanosterol (XXXIV), results from a series of directed oxidative cyclizations, with "activated molecular O_2" culminating in a hydroxylation at C-3 and the formation of four condensed rings with the migration of one carbon. These reactions comprise a striking example of the specificity of enzymes in directing specific ring closures and also specific methyl and hydrogen migration. The final transformation of lanosterol to cholesterol (III) includes the reduction of the 24-25 double bond, the migration of the 8-9 double bond to 5-6, and the oxidative removal of three methyl groups, two at C-4 and one at C-14. This overall mechanism virtually excludes the C_{18} or C_{21} steroids from being formed as intermediates in the biosynthesis of cholesterol, so that all the hormones appear to be derived from a common C_{27} and C_{30} precursor.

5.9   FROM CHOLESTEROL TO STEROID HORMONES

The series of steps from cholesterol (III) to pregnenolone (XXXVIII), not yet completely understood, is shown only in outline form in Figure 5.10. Cholesterol is first oxidized to the 20a-hydroxycholesterol (XXXV, XXXVI), then to 20a,22a--dihydroxycholesterol (XXXVII), and finally to pregnenolone and an isocaproic acid fragment. Alternative routes to 17a-hydroxypregnenolone via 17a,20a-dihydroxycholesterol have also been proposed. Pregnenolone (XXXVIII) is readily oxidized to progesterone (X), and either of these C_{21} derivatives is apparently the precursor of all other steroids produced in the adrenals, ovaries, and testes. This step of steroid biosynthesis is probably the most uncharted area remaining and could be extremely significant in the regulation of steroid-hormone biosynthesis and secretion. The conversion of cholesterol to the various steroid hormones has been studied in vivo and in gland perfusates, slices, and homogenates. These degradative reactions have a high tissue specificity. For example, the testes, adrenals, and placenta can convert cholesterol to pregnenolone and other derivatives but liver homogenates cannot. There is evidence that ACTH and the pituitary gonadotrophic hormones in the adrenals and gonads may be concerned with the desmolase reaction involving the rupture of the 20-22 carbon bond. Roberts *et al.* recently reported that c-AMP stimulated the conversion of cholesterol to pregnenolone in sonically disrupted adrenal mitochondria.

5.10   BIOSYNTHESIS OF THE ANDROGENS

The total biosynthesis of acetate to testosterone by a variety of pathways involving cholesterol and the C_{21} intermediates pregnenolone and progesterone occurs in the testes and several other steroid-producing tissues. The most prominent, well-identified routes to the androgens are summarized in Figure 5.11. These metabolic sequences reflect only a limited number of key steps. If pregnenolone has been the progenitor, they begin with hydroxylation at C-17, followed by oxidation at C-3; with progesterone as the precursor, the biogenesis need only involve 17a-

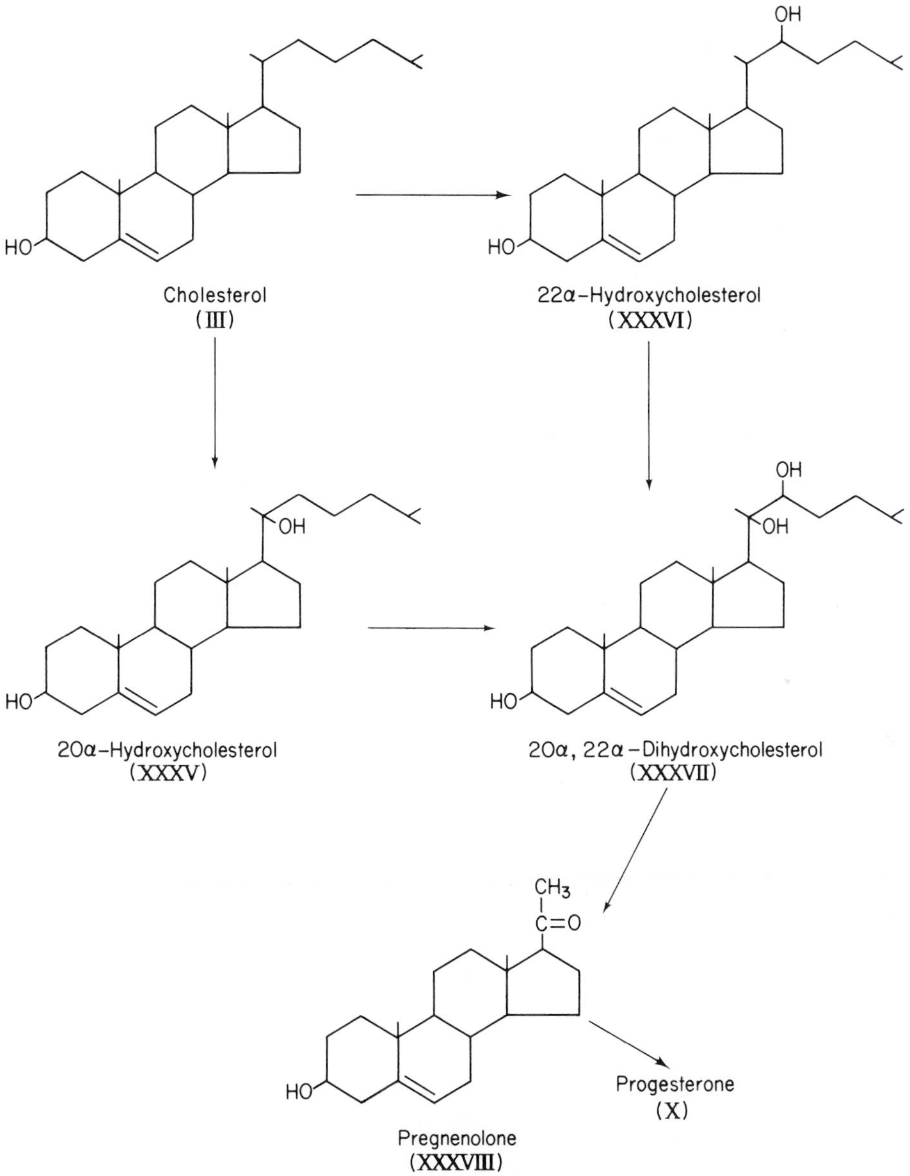

Figure 5.10 Conversion of cholesterol to pregnenolone.

hydroxyprogesterone and appropriate scission at C-17. Common intermediates or, in some cases, end-products such as androst-4-en-3,17-dione present no particular metabolic problem. These compounds are active in vivo and can be readily reduced by appropriate coupling with NADPH dehydrogenases.

Adrenal adenomas in vitro utilize dehydroepiandrosterone (see Figure 5.11) in a

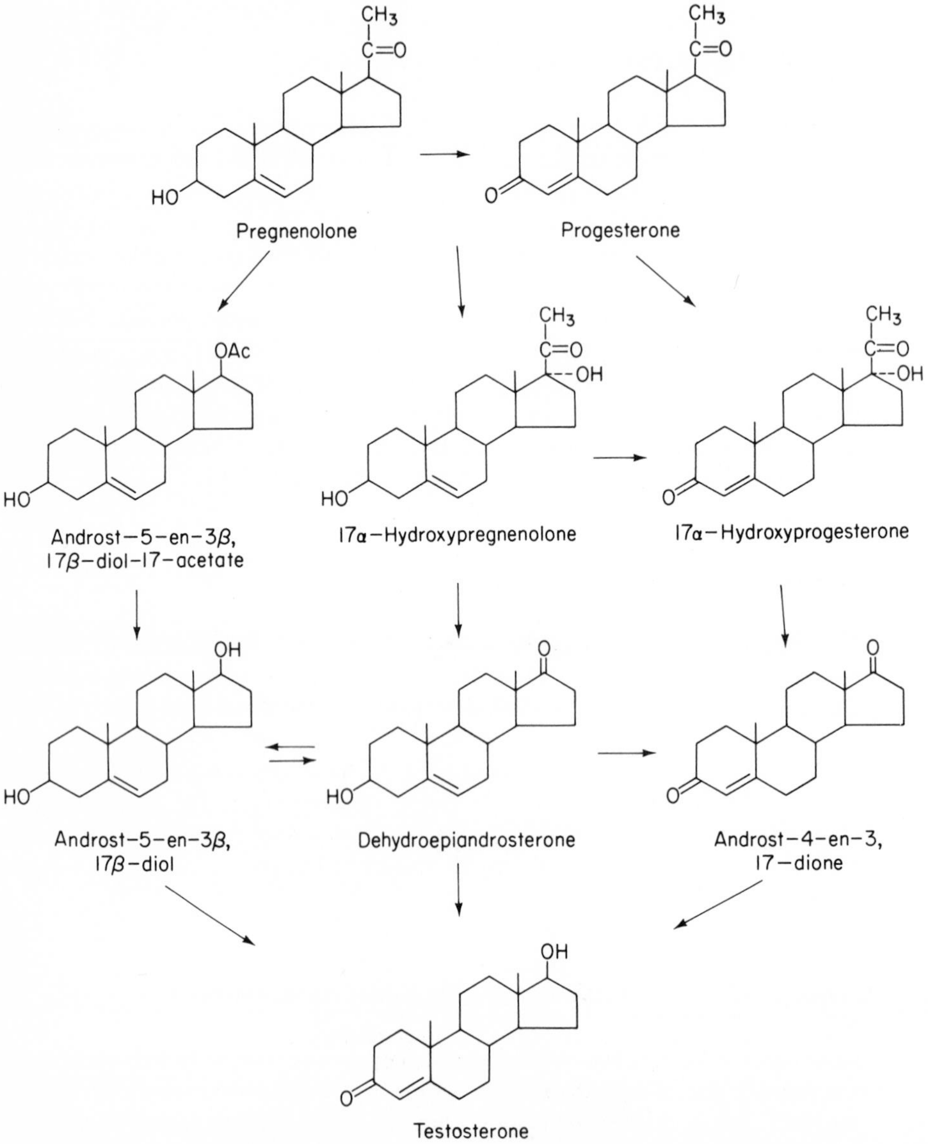

Figure 5.11 Biosynthetic pathways to the principal androgens.

common metabolic pathway; evidence for this pathway has been found in testes. Under certain conditions, adrenal tissue can convert almost any of the cortical steroids to C_{19} steroids having some degree of androgenic activity, as indicated by hirsutism or virilism in women with hyperactive adrenals. Finally, the possibility of direct formation of C_{19} steroids, without the necessity of a C_{21} intermediate, has also been suggested on the basis of isotopic studies, presumably involving a $17a,20a$-dihydroxycholesterol oxidation step.

5.11 BIOSYNTHESIS OF THE ESTROGENS

As early as 1934, in vivo studies suggested that estrogen formation proceeded primarily from androgens, and this was later confirmed with isotopic studies. Since they have identical functional groups, the problem of converting testosterone to estrone resolves itself to the elimination of the C-19 atom and the aromatization of ring A. Numerous tissues, including the ovary, placenta, and adrenals, have the ability to convert testosterone to estrogenic derivatives via 19-hydroxyandrost-4-en-3,17-dione. Ryan showed in 1959 that placental microsome preparations could convert 4-androsten-3,17-dione to estrone, in 50 to 60 percent yields. In addition to acetate, cholesterol, and progesterone, all the intermediate compounds shown in Figure 5.12 produce labeled estrone and estradiol. In the most direct path of the androgens to estrogen, the C-19 is successively oxidized to formaldehyde, followed by the loss of hydrogen from C-1 and C-2, and the enolization of C-3.

5.12 BIOSYNTHESIS OF THE ADRENAL STEROIDS

The adrenal steroids also originate from cholesterol via pregnenolone and progesterone. Hydroxylation of progesterone at C-21 yields 11-deoxycortico-sterone, one of the simplest structures with mineralcorticoid activity. Further hydroxylation at C-11, as shown in Figure 5.13, produces corticosterone; eventually, hydroxylation at C-17 yields cortisol (hydrocortisone). These key compounds also can be derived from pregnenolone and 17-hydroxypregnenolone. The biosynthesis of aldosterone utilizes several of the same intermediates as cortisol; however, intermediates 18,21-dihydroxyprogesterone and 18-hydroxycortico-sterone are unique to aldosterone biosynthesis.

5.13 METABOLISM AND EXCRETION OF THE STEROID HORMONES

Although the biosynthesis of the steroid hormones is now fairly well understood, the detailed fate of these compounds in the various peripheral tissues, particularly the liver, has only been partially elucidated. Three important general metabolic routes have been recognized: (1) conjugation or derivative formation; (2) hydrogenation of double bonds or keto groups; and (3) oxidation, especially at C-17.

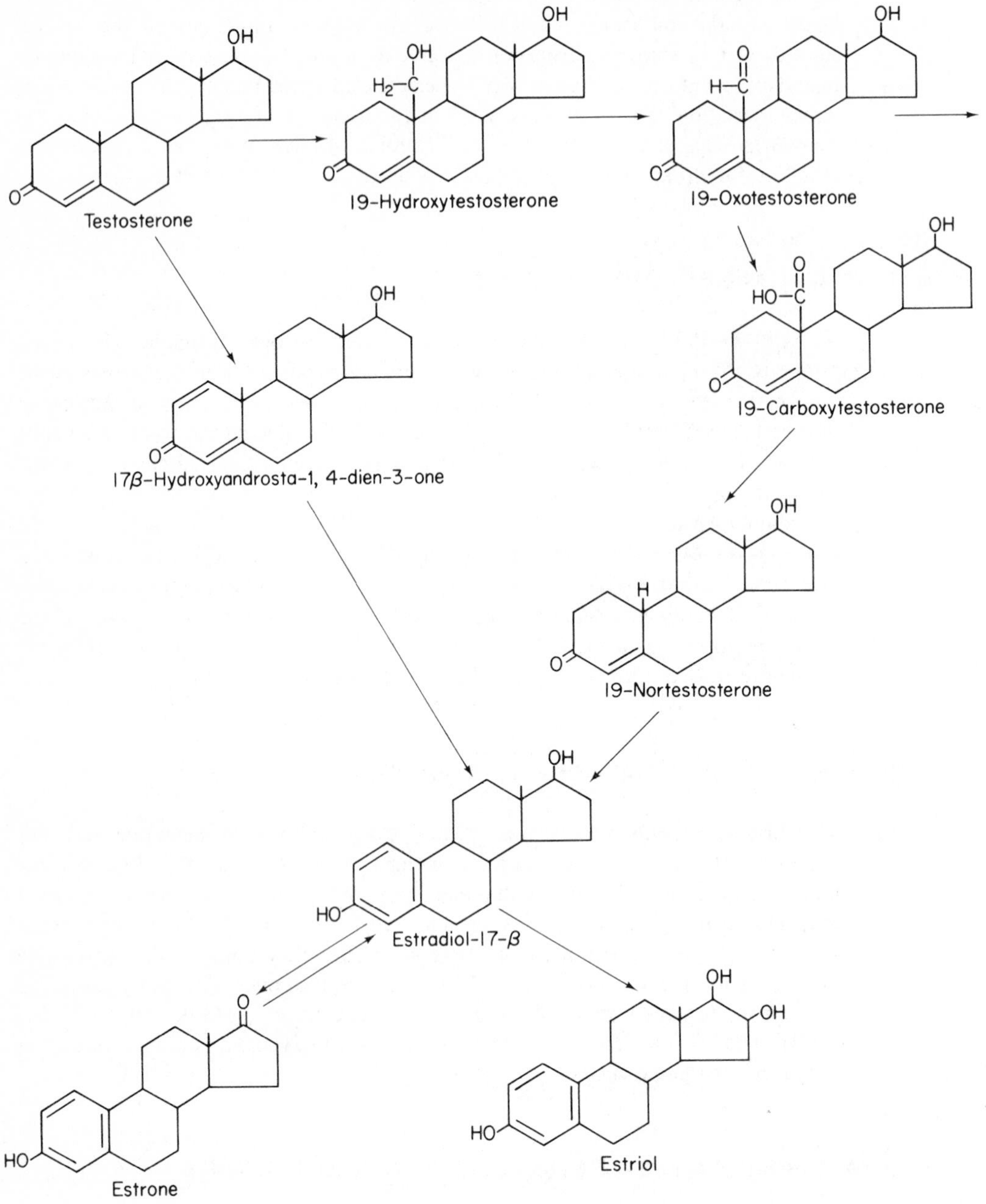

Figure 5.12 Biosynthetic pathways to the principal estrogens.

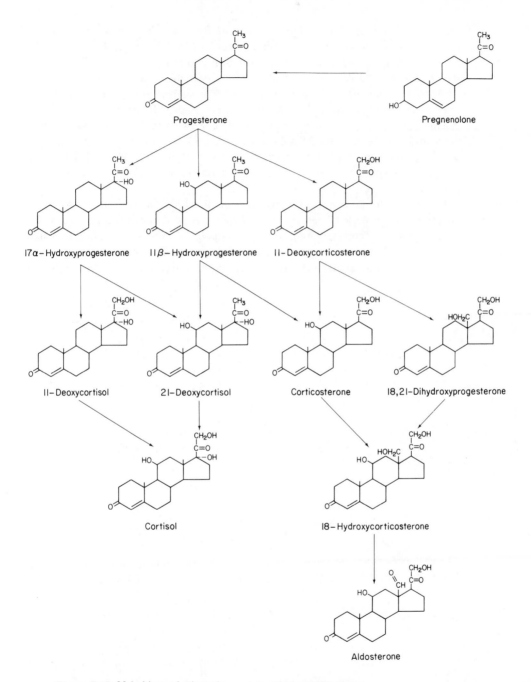

Figure 5.13 Main biosynthetic pathways to cortisol and aldosterone.

Complete oxidation of the steroid nucleus appears to be relatively rare. The first route involves glucuronide or sulfate ester formation, particularly with the hydroxyl group at C-3 or C-17, as indicated in two of the examples (XXXIX, XL) shown in Figure 5.14. This involves conversion of hydroxysteroids to water-soluble derivatives, which are more rapidly excreted. For analysis or isolation, these compounds are usually treated with appropriate hydrolytic enzymes, that is, β-glucuronidase and/or sulfatase. Many steroid hormones also undergo hydrogenation at the 4-5 double bond by Δ^4 reductases or at a 3α- or 3β-keto group by hydroxysteroid dehydrogenases; both of these reactions utilize NADH or NADPH. Examples of common reduced products are androsterone (XLI) and pregnanediol (XLII).

The metabolized steroids are excreted by the kidneys, with the consequent appearance of urinary 17-ketosteroids. These oxidized derivatives are generally less active than the corresponding parent compounds and arise from the many 17-hydroxy or 17-keto compounds, including estradiol, dehydroisoandrosterone, pregnanediol, and adrenal steroids. The 17-ketosteroids are frequently determined

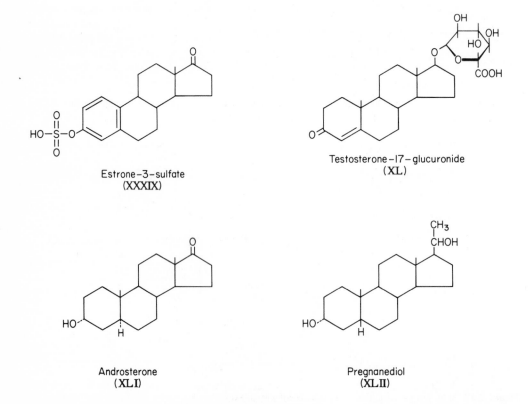

Estrone–3–sulfate
(XXXIX)

Testosterone–17–glucuronide
(XL)

Androsterone
(XLI)

Pregnanediol
(XLII)

Figure 5.14 Examples of steroid excretion products.

by the Zimmerman reaction, in which a purple color is formed after heating with 1,3-dinitrobenzene at alkaline pH values. The adult male excretes 8 to 30 mg of 17-ketosteroids daily; the normal adult female only 5 to 20 mg. A sharp threefold increase in production and excretion of 17-ketosteroids accompanies puberty. The quantity of 11-deoxy- and 11-oxy-17-ketosteroids provides an index of the relative secretory activities of the gonads and the adrenal cortex.

Certain diseases—for instance, adrenogenital syndrome (Cushing's disease) and tumors of the testes—are characterized by an increase in urinary 17-ketosteroids. The adrenogenital syndrome is due to an inborn error of metabolism in which the enzyme necessary for hydroxylation at C-21 is absent. Consequently 17-hydroxyprogesterone accumulates, cortisol formation is reduced, and feedback inhibition of ACTH secretion does not occur. Persistent stimulation by ACTH increases the output of adrenal steroids and the corresponding 17-ketosteroids. A normal level of steroid excretion can be restored by treatment with cortisol.

REFERENCES

Dorfman, R. I., and D. C. Sharma: "An Outline of the Biosynthesis of Cortico-steroids and Androgens," *Steroids,* **6,** 229 (1965).

Dorfman, R. I., and F. Ungar: *Metabolism and Steroid Hormones,* Academic Press, Inc., New York, 1965.

Fieser, L. F., and M. Fieser: *Steroids,* Reinhold Publishing Corp., New York, 1959.

SIX

THE SEX HORMONES

The gonads of each sex perform dual roles: (1) formation of gametes; (2) production of hormones that are responsible for growth and maintenance of the accessory sexual structures. In the male these structures include the gonadal ducts, seminal vesicles, coagulating gland, and prostate; in the female, fallopian tubes, uterus, vaginal epithelium, and mammary glands. In both sexes, these hormones are responsible for sexual behavior as well as body configuration.

The following description is generalized; it applies to mammals among whom some variation exists, but the variation is slight compared to that appearing among animals composing the rest of phylum Chordata.

6.1 EMBRYOLOGICAL DEVELOPMENT

The gonads of both sexes follow parallel pathways during their early embryological development: they originate from an area called the genital ridge in the vicinity of the future kidney or the dorsal wall of the embryonic body cavity. The genital ridge is composed of a layer of germinal epithelium and an internal epithelial mass.

The primordial germ cells originate in extraembryonic tissues and migrate, either by ameboid movement or through the blood stream, to the genital ridge. Testicular development involves greater development of the inner (medullary) portion of the gonad, while ovarian development is accompanied by greater development of the cortex. The primordial germ cells become surrounded by the germinal epithelium cells, which grow into the primary sex cords. If the gonads differentiate into a testis, the primary sex cords persist and form the seminiferous tubules while the primordial germ cells become spermatogonia. If the gonad differentiates into an ovary, the primary sex cords regress and a new growth of the cortex occurs, giving rise to secondary sex cords; the primary germ cells then multiply and become oogonia. The oogonia become surrounded by follicle cells, possibly from the secondary sex cords. The follicles (with their contained oogonia) number about 200,000 to 300,000 in each ovary at birth. Additional oogonia do not arise in the ovaries during the life of the organism.

6.2 ANATOMY OF THE MALE AND FEMALE

The testes are present as paired organs in the male of most vertebrate species. They are composed of very long seminiferous tubules, which are lined by spermatogonia, Sertoli cells, and sperm in various stages of development [that is, primary spermatocytes, secondary spermatocytes (haploid), spermatids, and mature sperm]. The heads of the sperm cells are imbedded in the Sertoli cells, where they complete their maturation. Outside the seminiferous tubules are masses of cells, the interstitial or Leydig cells, which are the source of the androgens and estrogens secreted by the testes.

In the majority of mammals, the testes descend into the scrotum, at least during the breeding season. In a small number of species, the testes remain in the abdomen throughout life, for example, the duckbill, spiny anteater, sloth, armadillo, dugong, elephant, whale, and dolphin. In other species, these organs may be located in either the inguinal canal or the perineum, or they may appear periodically or permanently in the scrotum. Retention of the testes in the body cavity of animals that normally have descended testes is called cryptorchidism. This condition is simulated if descended testes are returned to the body cavity; degeneration of testicular epithelium then occurs, with failure of spermatogenesis and reduced testosterone synthesis. The scrotum serves as a thermoregulatory structure, maintaining the temperature of the testes at 1 to $3°C$ cooler than the body temperature. Two sets of muscles are involved in the thermoregulatory reflex: one set, the cremaster muscles, attaches to the testes; the other set, the tunica dartos, inserts into the skin of the scrotum. Cooling the body causes both sets of muscles to contract, pulling the testes close to the body.

The ovaries are suspended from the dorsal wall of the body cavity and frequently are contained in the lower half of the abdomen. Although they usually develop as paired organs, only the left ovary develops in birds, and in some mammalian species (such as duckbills and bats) only one ovary is functional. The ovaries are composed of follicles in various stages of development, ranging from primary to mature (Graafian) follicles. Distributed among the follicles is the interstitial tissue; the amount of this tissue varies according to species. In adult female mammals, the ovary also contains degenerating follicles, atretic follicles, corpora lutea (formed after ovulation), and corpora albicans (the residue of degenerated corpora lutea).

6.3 ACTION OF THE SEX HORMONES

Androgens

Sex hormones exert an effect on differentiation of the embryonic gonad. In susceptible species, estrogens cause sex reversal of the male with formation of an ovotestes or even complete feminization. Androgens also cause sex reversal of the female, with altered development ranging from the formation of an ovotestes through complete transformation to a male. Although the testes are the primary source of testosterone, dehydroepiandrosterone, and androstenediene, the adrenals also synthesize and secrete small amounts of these substances. Androgens have a specific function in the maintenance of the testes, reproductive tract, and secondary sexual characteristics of the male. Testosterone is necessary for spermatogenesis, continued function of the reproductive-tract glands, growth of the testes and scrotum, growth and distribution of body hair, body configuration, secondary masculine structures of birds, amphibia, and fish, and male aggressive behavior.

Metabolically, androgens stimulate protein metabolism and induce positive nitrogen balance. Castration in prepuberal animals results in failure of the reproductive tract to mature and failure of secondary sexual characteristics to appear. Castration after puberty causes regression and atrophy of the structures of the reproductive tract and secondary sexual characteristics. Testosterone allows normal development in the prepuberal castrate and maintenance of masculine characteristics and structure in the postpuberal castrate (eunuch).

Androgens exert effects on widely diverse tissues. They affect sex-specific tissues such as the penis, ventral prostate, and seminal vesicles of mammals and the comb, wattles, and spur of the cock. These hormones also exert effects on other organs such as the kidney and liver. They increase activities of β-glucuronidase, arginase, esterase, and D-amino acid oxidase in the kidney and activity of aldolase in the rat ventral prostate. In the liver, the microsomal content of NADPH oxidase is increased by testosterone.

The ability of testosterone to induce protein synthesis in muscle as well as other tissues has led to a more detailed analysis of its action. Testosterone treatment increases protein synthesis by ribosomes from castrated rat muscle. This action of testosterone is inhibited by actinomycin D. Thus, testosterone may exert its effect either in the nucleus, by increasing RNA polymerase activity (affecting transcriptional control) or on the mRNA-ribosomal complex (affecting translational control); see Chapter 10, pages 150-151.

Estrogens

Estrogens are produced during follicular growth by steroid secreting cells among the fibroblasts of the theca interna; during the luteal phase of ovarian cycles, they are produced along with progesterone by the corpus luteum. In the horse, the corpus luteum contains two cell populations responsible for secretion of both steroids. The extremely high concentrations of estrogens, found in the urine of stallions, are assumed to come from the testes since little estrogen appears in the urine of geldings. Estrogens have also been found in the urine of normal men, the amount excreted increasing after administration of HCG. Estrogen secretion by the ovary is under the control of the pituitary hormones. Neither FSH nor LH alone can stimulate sufficient estrogen secretion to maintain the uterine weight in hypophysectomized rats but FSH and LH together are effective when administered over a wide range of ratios of hormones.

Estrogens act on the adult ovary, causing hypertrophy of the follicle granulosa in hypophysectomized rats. These hormones act on the hypothalamus to inhibit LH secretion (see Chapter 2) and on the pituitary to inhibit LH secretion; also, they are necessary for the development of the gonadoduct system in the female organism. The action of estrogens on the uterus has been correlated with an estrogen-chromatin complex in the nuclei, an increase in synthesis of ribosomal RNA, an increased rate of formation of ribosomal precursor particles, and the transport of RNA to the cytoplasm. Estrogens may affect uterine protein synthesis by an action at the transcriptional level, but estrogen-induced increases in RNA synthesis have been shown to depend upon prior protein synthesis—suggesting that there is a protein synthesis (presently undefined) which precedes RNA synthesis. The mechanism of action of estrogens on the uterus may be similar to that of their action on other susceptible tissues such as the mammary gland, and beak and plumage in birds.

Progestins

Coitus, LH, or HCG causes ovulation in the rabbit in 10 to 12 hr. The ruptured follicle is then transformed into a corpus luteum. Shortly after the original stimulus, secretion of 20a-hydroxypregn-4-en-3-one from the interstitial tissue begins, persisting for about 6 hr; in spayed, mated females, this substance sustains adenohypophyseal LH secretion. Hilliard has suggested that this progestin, synthesized and secreted under the influence of LH, acts as a positive-feedback control to prolong the LH secretion. Although LH is normally secreted in the rabbit for about 6 hr, and has a half-life in the circulation of only 22 min, ovulation does occur if hypophysectomy is performed one hour after mating. Therefore, LH either persists in the ovary for a long time or within a few hours of exposure it initiates changes in this tissue that continue after the hormone is undetectable in the blood and that lead to ovulation. If actinomycin D, puromycin, or cycloheximide is injected into the mature follicles of mated rabbits, only those follicles that receive the drugs within 4 hr after mating fail to ovulate (Figure 6.1). The interpretation

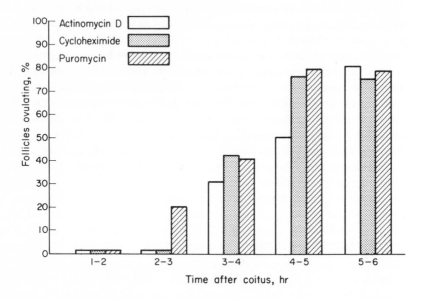

Figure 6.1   The effect of inhibitors of transcription (actinomycin D) and of translation (cycloheximide and puromycin) on ovulation of rabbit Graafian follicles. The inhibitory solutions were injected directly into rabbit Graafian follicles at various intervals after mating in volumes of 1 μl. The concentration of actinomycin D was 0.001 μg/ml; that of the cycloheximide and puromycin was 1 μg/μl. The inhibitory compounds were controlled by saline injection into adjacent follicles on the same ovary. Inhibitors were ineffective when introduced more than 4 hr after mating.

Time, hr	Animals, Total Number			Follicles, Total Number			$p^b < 0.01$		
	AMD[a]	CH[a]	PM[a]	AMD	CH	PM	AMD	CH	PM
1-2	4	4	3	9	21	8	*	*	*
2-3	4	3	4	11	20	15	*	*	*
3-4	2	2	4	14	13	14	*		
4-5	2	3	5	4	12	14			
5-6	3	2	6	5	14	13			

[a]AMD, actinomycin D; CH, cycloheximide; PM, puromycin.

[b]The probability that the observation is due to chance is less than 1 percent.

[c]The * indicates the conditions under which significant differences were found.

[Data from W. R. Pool and H. Lipner, "Inhibition of Ovulation in the Rabbit by Actinomycin D," *Nature,* **203,** 1385 (1964), and "Inhibition of Ovulation by Antibiotics," *Endocrinol.,* **79,** 858 (1966).]

that ovulation is preceded by RNA and protein synthesis is also supported by the radioautographic observation that H^3-uridine and H^3-valine are incorporated into the two inner layers of the follicle wall before ovulation.

The ruptured follicle is transformed into a corpus luteum by the action of LH; however, luteinization of follicles can occur after large doses of LH or HCG without rupture of the follicle. Continued functioning of the corpus luteum of the estrous cycle (as contrasted with the corpus luteum of pregnancy) may be either dependent on adenohypophyseal secretion of luteotrophic factors or independent of subsequent extrinsic stimuli. In rodents, prolactin is luteotrophic; in cows, pigs, and humans, LH is the luteotrophic hormone, but in sheep, rabbits, and pigs, estradiol allows a normal life span for the corpus luteum after hypophysectomy. In animals with short estrous cycles (rats and mice), the corpus luteum produces insufficient amounts of progesterone to induce a decidual reaction [hypertrophy of the superficial layer of the uterine wall (endometrium) and hyperplasia of the endometrial stroma], the change in the uterus preceding implantation of a fertilized egg. Progesterone must act on the uterus for 48 hr in order for a decidual reaction to occur.

The progestin predominantly formed by the corpus luteum is progesterone. Administration of LH causes an increase within bovine corpora lutea of adenylcyclase formation with consequent increased phosphorylase activity, utilization of glucose, and synthesis of progesterone. Steroidogenesis and synthesis of progesterone can also be stimulated by c-AMP, its dibutaryl analog, or theophylline. Savard suggested that the second-messenger mechanism of c-AMP for control of steroidogenesis involves the synthesis of cholesterol precursors. An alternative interpretation, suggested by Armstrong and Greep, is that LH accelerates the conversion of cholesterol to progesterone and that c-AMP has no effect on this conversion.

An extension of the latter hypothesis emphasizes that the rat corpus luteum produces 20α-hydroxypregn-4-en-3-one under the influence of LH. This steroid—which exerts 1/25 of the progestational effect of progesterone—is formed as a result of the induction of 20α-hydroxysteroid dehydrogenase by LH. Prolactin inhibits its induction and causes progesterone to become the end-product of steroid biosynthesis in the corpus luteum.

The uterus in guinea pigs, sheep, and pigs apparently exerts a luteotrophic effect on the corpus luteum for approximately the first two-thirds of the life of the corpus luteum, and a luteolytic effect after this period. The corpus luteum persists very much longer in hysterectomized guinea pigs. The formation of progesterone is stimulated by extracts prepared from guinea-pig uteri with young corpora lutea and inhibited by extracts prepared from uteri obtained with old corpora lutea. Such phenomena in guinea pigs, sheep, pigs, and cows led workers to suggest that the uterus is the source of a luteolytic factor.

Progesterone plays a number of important roles in the reproductive life of mammals. It speeds the movement of the ovum through the fallopian tubes, prepares the uterine endometrium for implantation, and inhibits contractility of the uterine myometrium, thus allowing pregnancy to continue; in the absence of progesterone, pregnancies quickly terminate. It is also essential for the development of the mammary glands: in the presence of estrogens, which cause duct growth, progesterone causes the development of the glandular portions, the alveoli. However, production of milk requires prolactin as well as ACTH, GH, and thyroid hormone (see Chapter 2).

Relaxin

A third sex hormone, relaxin, has been found in the corpus luteum, placenta, and uterus. Relaxin is a polypeptide with a molecular weight of about 9,000. It is most effective in animals with high concentrations of circulatory estrogen and progesterone (during estrus or pregnancy). Relaxin causes the ligaments of the symphis pubis of guinea pigs and mice to increase in distensibility, and increases dilation of the cervix in pregnant women at parturition. It synergizes with progesterone and estrogen to maintain gestation, and its concentrations decline rapidly several days prior to parturition.

6.4 CYCLIC REGULATION OF REPRODUCTION

Reproductive periods may be classified into seasonal and continuous estrous cycles. The estrous cycle is the period between recurring stages of sexual receptivity, which are usually called heat or estrus. Cycles may be monoestrous (occurring once per year) or polyestrous (occurring two or more times per year). Continuous estrous cycles have a duration that is species-specific; for example, the cycle lasts from 4 to 5 days in the rat, up to 16 days in the guinea pig and ewe, and up to 21 days in the cow and sow. A further modification in cyclic mechanism is the separation of continuously cycling species into spontaneous ovulators (for example, cow, sow, ewe, and guinea pig) and induced ovulators (such as rabbit, mink, cat, and ferret). The spontaneous ovulator has an estrous time that coincides with the initiation of ovulation, whereas the induced ovulator is receptive to a male at any time, and ovulates at a variable time after coitus: after mating, the rabbit ovulates in 10 hr, the cat in 24 hr, and the ferret in 30 hr. Ovulation is due to the barrage of stimuli acting on the hypothalamus, generating the release of FRH and LRH, which cause the secretion of pituitary gonadotrophins (see Figure 2.9).

Spontaneous rhythmical sexual activity of the female, although more difficult to explain, has been carefully explored in the rat. Gorski and Wagner have summarized their own work and that of others to formulate a hypothesis based on hypothalamic regulation of the secretion of gonadotrophin-releasing hormone (Figure 6.2). They have assumed that the anterior hypothalamus and preoptic areas are undifferentiated but are inherently cyclic (intermittent) regulators of LH secretion and that the ventromedial and arcuate nuclei are inherently tonic (constant) regulators of gonadotrophin secretion. From the first day to the fifth day after birth, the anterior hypothalamus and preoptic areas can respond to endogenous or exogenous testosterone propionate or estradiol benzoate. Treatment of a neonatal female with either of these substances or by transplantation of testes causes

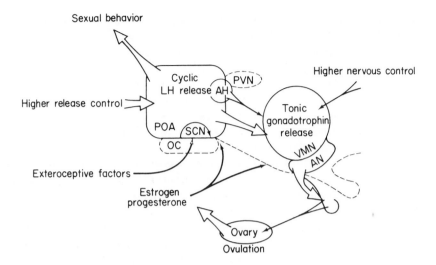

Figure 6.2   Diagrammatic representation of the localization of gonadotrophin-regulating mechanisms within the hypothalamus of the female rat. Abbreviations: AH, anterior hypothalamus; AN, arcuate nucleus; OC, optic chiasma; POA, preoptic area; PVN, paraventricular nucleus; SCN, suprachiasmatic nucleus; VMN, ventromedial nucleus. [Reprinted from R. A. Gorski, "Localization and Sexual Differentiation of the Nervous Structures which Regulate Ovulation," *J. Reprod. Fert. Suppl.,* **1,** 67-88 (1966).]

entrance into continuous estrus at puberty and enlargement of many ovarian follicles. Castration of neonatal males results in the appearance of corpora lutea in subsequent ovarian transplants. These two experimental situations are indicative of reversal of the neural pattern and of its lability. They also indicate that the nervous system of the neonatal female is neutral and that testosterone exerts a positive effect by causing the nervous system to differentiate in a subtle manner that becomes apparent only after puberty.

The estrous cycle may be divided into two general phases: (1) *follicular phase,* the period of follicle growth and maturation, marked by increasing secretion of estrogen and changes in the uterine and vaginal mucosa; (2) the *luteal phase,* initiated by ovulation of the follicle and its subsequent conversion to a corpus luteum. The duration of the luteal phase depends upon whether or not the corpus luteum becomes functional and secretes progesterone, with its consequent effect upon the uterine and vaginal mucosa. The phases of ovarian function have been divided into stages initially described by Stockard and Papanicolau; these phases are correlated with the cytology of the vagina. In the rat, the smears of the vaginal wall reveal a changing pattern of cells and mucus. In early estrus, the smear is composed almost exclusively of cornified epithelial cells. Later in estrus, much mucus appears in the vaginal smear while the cornified cells are still very prominent. A smear taken 12 hr later, during metestrus, contains cornified cells, many leucocytes, and almost no mucus. In the rat, cycles follow each other quickly: the corpora lutea are nonsecretory and metestrus is brief unless pregnancy or pseudopregnancy ensues. In animals with secretory corpora lutea, metestrus is prolonged. Diestrus is associated with a vaginal smear containing almost only leucocytes and occasional oval-shaped cells with large nuclei, nucleated epithelial cells. One day later, the vaginal smear is characterized by only the nucleated epithelial cells; the animal is then in proestrus. Diestrus, proestrus, and estrus occur during the follicular phase of ovarian function, whereas metestrus occurs during the luteal phase. Knowledge of the relationship between vaginal cytology and ovarian function has provided physiologists and biochemists with a powerful experimental tool.

In primates, the reproductive cycle is the *menstrual cycle*, which extends from the first day of bleeding to the day before the next bleeding period begins. Rhesus monkeys and women have cycle durations with a mode of 28 days and an average of 33 ± 0.6 days. Ovulation is spontaneous, occurring approximately in midcycle (between the eleventh and fourteenth days). Primates are sexually receptive throughout the cycle; they therefore have no estrus stage during the menstrual cycle. The menstrual cycle also can be divided into follicular and luteal phases. During the follicular phase the uterine endometrium grows thicker and the glandular structure elongates into tubes with spiral arteries distributed throughout the endometrium. The luteal phase is characterized by increased tortuosity of the spiral arteries and by secretory activity of the endometrial glands. Menstruation occurs when the corpus luteum stops secreting progesterone. Bleeding from the spiral arteries and sloughing of the endometrium persists for 3 to 5 days, followed by a new growth of the endometrium.

A number of behavioral, morphological, and functional changes are associated with estrus in nonprimates and with ovulation in primates. Rats, rabbits, and most nonprimates in estrus become passive in the presence of males: shortly after being mounted, the female depresses her abdomen toward the ground and rotates her pelvis upward in a lordosis. Female animals increase their physical activity: rats run more in activity cages, and women walk more. The vaginal mucus becomes more fluid, forms fernlike patterns on drying, and is more acidic. The basal body temperature of women declines about 0.6°C on the morning of ovulation and then rises slowly about 0.7°C until menstruation, when the cycle begins again. Their sensitivity to cold increases with the sharp decline in basal body temperature.

6.5 ENDOCRINOLOGY OF PREGNANCY AND PARTURITION

The relationship of the adenohypophysis and the ovary to the continuation of pregnancy is seen in Table 6.1. Animals such as mice and rats can maintain a pregnancy to term if hypophysectomized after midpregnancy (day 11) but abort after ovariectomy. In these animals, the placenta may be the source of a luteotrophin that maintains the activity of the corpus luteum. In animals such as sheep, guinea pigs, Rhesus monkeys, and humans, in which hypophysectomy and ovariectomy do not terminate pregnancy, the placenta is the source of progesterone; either its secretion is independent of luteotrophic factors or these are also formed in the placenta. In man, the placenta is the source of HCG, which acts on the corpus luteum to maintain progesterone secretion. In guinea pigs, sheep, cattle, horses, and humans, the placenta is also a source of progesterone; sufficient amounts are produced to maintain pregnancy during the latter part of the gestation period in the absence of both the adenohypophysis and the ovaries.

The length of the gestation period is species-dependent: for example, in the rat it is about 21 days and in the elephant it is 624 days. The factors that cause parturition are variable and also species-dependent. Progesterone can prolong gestation in rats and rabbits, but in cows, sheep, Rhesus monkeys, humans, horses, and guinea pigs, progesterone does not delay parturition. Estrogens sensitize the uteri of rats, mice, rabbits, and cats to oxytocin, and can cause abortion in these species. In a number of species, for example, humans, rabbits, and guinea pigs, oxytocin causes parturition, supporting the hypothesis that oxytocin is involved in determining the length of the gestation period. Another hypothesis suggests that in rabbits and humans, the volume of the uterus exerts an effect on placental secretion of progesterone, and local concentrations of progesterone determine the spontaneous contractility of uterine smooth muscle. In sheep the mean length of the gestation period is 151 days. Hypophysectomy of fetal lambs between days 93 and 143 of gestation results in prolongation of pregnancy; ACTH administered to hypophysectomized fetal lambs causes parturition but is ineffective when given to hypophysectomized and adrenalectomized fetal lambs. The fetal hypophyseal-adrenal axis is involved in the induction of parturition, therefore the hypothalamic-hypophyseal mechanism must also be active. Other factors that may influence the duration of the gestation period (and even affect the activity of the uterine myometrium) are sex of the fetus, fetal genotype, and presence of a fetal hypophysis.

TABLE 6.1 COMPARISON OF THE EFFECTS OF HYPOPHYSECTOMY AND OF OVARIECTOMY IN DIFFERENT MAMMALIAN SPECIES[a]

Species	Effect[b]		Earliest date[c]	
	Hypophysectomy	Ovariectomy	Hypophysectomy	Ovariectomy
Rabbit	Aborted	Aborted	Near term	Near Term
Dog	Aborted	Continued	Near term	Day 30 (?)
Guinea pig	Continued	Continued	Day 40–41	Day 20
Mouse	Continued	Absorbed, aborted	Day 10	—
Rat	Continued	Absorbed, aborted	Day 11	—
Sheep	Continued	Continued	Day 50	Day 54
Rhesus monkey	Continued	Continued	Day 27	Day 25
Man	Continued	Continued	Week 12	Day 30

[a]From A. Van Tienhoven, *Reproductive Physiology of Vertebrates*, p. 336, W. B. Saunders Co., Philadelphia, 1968.

[b]Effect of hypophysectomy or ovariectomy is indicated as either *aborted* or *absorbed* if the operation caused these effects at any time during pregnancy except close to term, or as *continued* if pregnancy was not interrupted after the operation.

[c]Earliest date at which the operation was compatible with maintenance of pregnancy.

REFERENCES

Asdell, S. A.: *Patterns of Mammalian Reproduction*, 2nd ed., Cornell University Press, Ithaca, N. Y., 1964.

van Tienhoven, Ari: *Reproductive Physiology of Vertebrates*, W. B. Saunders Co., Philadelphia, 1968.

Young, W. C.: *Sex and Internal Secretions*, 3rd ed., vols. 1 and 2, The Williams & Wilkins Co., Baltimore, 1961.

Zuckerman, S.: *The Ovary*, Academic Press, Inc., New York, 1962.

SEVEN

THE ADRENAL HORMONES

7.1 THE ADRENAL CORTEX

The adrenal gland is divided into three outer layers of cortical tissue, which secrete 40 to 50 steroids, and an inner medulla responsible for the biosynthesis of epinephrine. In higher vertebrates, the adrenal glands are oval masses embedded in fatty tissue resting near the anterior pole of the kidney. In some lower vertebrates, the cortex and medulla may exist independently, distributed along blood vessels in the lower abdomen.

The cells of the adrenal cortex develop from the embryonic mesoderm into three discernible layers. Under the capsule that envelops the gland is a thin cortical layer, the *zona glomerulosa*. This layer consists of columnar cells responsible for the synthesis and secretion of aldosterone and is relatively uninfluenced by ACTH. The lack of a sharp separation between the effects of ACTH on glucocorticoid and mineralcorticoid secretion probably arises from the fact that the glucocorticoids possess appreciable sodium-retention activity, particularly in view of the much higher daily output in man of cortisol (25 mg/day) and corticosterone

111

(5 mg/day) in contrast to aldosterone (0.25 mg/day). The next layer of cells, the *zona fasciculata,* gradually merges into the *zona reticularis,* which surrounds the medulla and is clearly demarcated from it. The cells of the two inner cortex layers synthesize glucocorticoids under the control of ACTH, a typical example of a negative-feedback-control system. The rates of secretion of cortisol, corticosterone, and most of the other adrenal steroids are determined by variations in the release of ACTH from the pituitary (see Figure 2.8). Incubation of adrenal tissue with ACTH results in an increased release of cortical steroids and a marked reduction of ascorbic acid. The latter response is the basis of a classical bioassay for ACTH as developed by Sayers *et al.* (More recent test methods include the release of corticoids into the adrenal vein of the hypophysectomized rat and an immunochemical test for plasma ACTH.) ACTH is required for the maintenance of responsive portions of the adrenals: after hypophysectomy the zona fasciculata and zona reticularis atrophy, whereas the glomerulosa hypertrophies.

7.2 EFFECT OF ADRENALECTOMY—THE STRESS REACTION

Removal of the adrenal glands dramatically affects the metabolism of experimental animals. The adrenal steroids are the family of hormones that permit the animal to make a long-term adjustment to metabolic stress. Adrenalectomized animals survive only if NaCl and food are freely available and no significant environmental or physiological challenges are presented (for example, suboptimal temperatures or trauma). An early response of normal animals exposed to stress is increased adrenocortical secretion, indicated by involution of the thymus and eosinopenia. Under the influence of cortical steroids, the animal can adapt to the new stress and survive until his physiological defense mechanisms are exhausted or until the stress subsides. Selye has termed this entire phenomenon the "general adaptation" syndrome.

The most crucial metabolic disturbance after adrenalectomy is the inability to retain Na, leading to a spectrum of ion and water imbalances arising from loss of water from the circulation. The changes in the blood include increased erythrocyte count, most easily seen by the increase in the hematocrit, reduced plasma volume and blood flow, and a two- to threefold increase in serum urea and serum potassium. The loss of sodium causes a drop in the osmotic pressure of the body fluids, with a profound disruption of electrolyte and water balance. Plasma Na^+ and K^+ are maintained at normal concentrations in the adrenalectomized dog with 10 μg aldosterone/day, whereas 5,000 μg cortisol/day is required to achieve normal concentrations of these ions. The effect of aldosterone can be detected within 30 to 90 min and lasts 4 to 8 hr, stimulating renal reabsorption of Na^+ H^+, NH_4^+, and Mg^{2+}; it also increases water absorption (as a result of Na^+ retention). After adrenalectomy, significant changes in electrolyte balance are observed within 1 day following withdrawal of replacement steroids. Later, a fall in plasma volume, blood flow, body temperature, O_2 uptake, and blood pressure is accompanied by an increase in blood urea and plasma proteins. Ultimately, these disturbances are responsible for the death of the animal. Adrenalectomized animals survive if fed 0.9 percent NaCl solution instead of water. Such animals, however, are unable to adapt to any major chemical or physical stress, and cannot tolerate temperature extremes, starvation, infection, sensitizing agents, and noxious chemicals. Appropriate doses of aldosterone, deoxycorticosterone, and other mineralcorticoids can replace the need for high intake of sodium. This syndrome is observable in patients with adrenal insufficiency (Addison's disease). In typical Addison's disease, maximal reabsorption of Na is reduced from 99.5 to 98.5 percent, with a consequent loss of about 6 g Na/day. Other effects arising from increased Na excretion and K retention include muscular weakness, acidosis, hypotension, and decreased cardiac output.

Maintenance of adrenalectomized animals in an adequate salt balance allows the important role of the glucocorticoids in the metabolism of carbohydrates and proteins to become apparent. The relationship of glucocorticoids to the metabolic effects of insulin was recognized by Houssay (in 1930) when he showed that the precarious metabolic balance of the depancreatized dog could be stabilized if the dog were simultaneously hypophysectomized (the "Houssay animal"). Later, in 1936, Long showed that adrenalectomy had a similar effect on pancreatectomized cats (the "Long cat").

7.3 CONTROL OF ADRENAL STEROID SECRETION

The secretion of the glucocorticoids is under the control of ACTH (see Chapter 2, pages 27-30). The glucocorticoids produced as a result of the action of ACTH exert a negative-feedback control on the hypothalamus to inhibit the release of CRH with consequent reduction of ACTH secretion by the adenohypophysis. Control of the secretion of aldosterone by the zona glomerulosa involves a different regulatory mechanism, as shown in Figure 7.1. The primary event in this regulatory mechanism in humans and dogs, where it has been studied extensively, is the stimulation of renin secretion by the kidney under conditions of a declining blood volume or pressure or decreased Na^+ concentration. Renin causes cleavage of a decapeptide, angiotensin I, from angiotensinogen (a plasma α_2-globulin having a molecular weight of 30,000). A converting enzyme present in plasma hydrolyzes angiotensin I to an octapeptide, angiotensin II. It is angiotensin II that exerts the stimulus on the adrenal cortex that induces aldosterone secretion; ACTH and K^+ also induce the secretion of aldosterone. However, the response to angiotensin II is greater and its effect is potentiated in the presence of ACTH and K^+ at concentrations of angiotensin II that are otherwise ineffective (see Figure 9.3, page 136).

7.4 EFFECT OF THE ADRENAL STEROIDS

Interest in corticoid-hormone action came with the recognition that adrenal tumors secrete excess steroids. The pathology encountered as a result of these lesions depends on the steroid(s) produced by the tumor. In Cushing's disease (adrenogenital syndrome), the predominant steroid is cortisol. The effect of the excess glucocorticoids include marked localized fat deposits (e.g., buffalo humpback or moonface), muscular weakness, disturbances in electrolyte balance, hypertension, and frequently diabetes. If the predominant steroid produced by the tumor is aldosterone, extensive disturbances of salt distribution result in edema, hypertension, cardiac failure, and extreme muscular weakness. In some instances, hypersecretion of steroids with androgenic activity leads to adrenal virilism in women and precocious sexual development in children. The masculinization process in the adult is accompanied by growth of the beard (hirsutism), atrophy of the breasts, and inhibition of ovulation. Removal of the adrenals and the tumor must be followed by replacement therapy with natural or synthetic glucocorticoids (see Chapter 5, page 87).

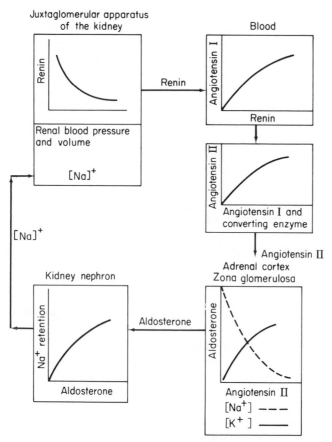

Figure 7.1   Regulation of the secretion of aldosterone is achieved by the action of angiotensin II on the adrenal cortex. Aldosterone causes an increase in sodium retention. The sodium ion concentration determines the secretion of renin by the juxtaglomerular apparatus and may affect the conversion of corticosterone to aldosterone by increasing the activity of the 18-hydroxy-dehydrogenase when present in low concentrations. The amount of sodium retained also regulates the blood pressure and volume.

The discovery by Hench and co-workers (in 1949) of the remarkable therapeutic effects of the glucocorticoids on a bewildering variety of metabolic diseases for which few other remedies were available stimulated an enormous amount of clinical and basic research on ACTH and the glucocorticoids. The disorders affected include rheumatoid arthritis, rheumatic fever, hypersensitivity, and many acute inflammatory and allergic diseases. This most useful therapy is a striking example of the productivity of endocrine research, since the original clue for this discovery came from a careful study of the improvement of a variety of metabolic diseases during human pregnancy.

7.5 MECHANISM OF ACTION OF THE ADRENAL STEROIDS

Mineralcorticoids

The basis for aldosterone action in regulating Na and K balance has been the subject of recent intensive efforts of several research groups. Edelman and associates have reported that aldosterone is preferentially absorbed by kidney nuclei, where it triggers the synthesis of selected mRNA's, which in turn lead to increased mitochondrial oxidative-enzyme assemblies and greater ATP generation via oxidative phosphorylation. Evidence for an aldosterone-induced protein synthesis is in part based upon inhibition of kidney tubule transport by actinomycin D, puromycin, cycloheximide, and amino acid antagonists (ethionine, p-fluorophenylalanine, and so forth). The greater availability of ATP at the site of the sodium pump leads to increased Na reabsorption from the kidney ultrafiltrate by increasing the rate of Na transport through the epithelial cells. Membrane-bound adenosine triphosphatase also may be involved in the regulation of the sodium pump. Sharp and Leaf favor the idea of a more direct effect of aldosterone on the transport process, perhaps through the enhanced synthesis of a specific permease protein that facilitates the movement of Na^+ through the mucosal surface.

Glucocorticoids

Most of the metabolic actions of adrenocortical extracts have been attributed to the effect of the glucocorticoids. The term *glucocorticoid* arose in defining the action of the C_{21} steroids (with hydroxyl groups at C-11 and C-17) that maintain normal blood sugar and liver glycogen levels in adrenalectomized animals (see Figure 5.6 for details of the chemical structure of these steroids). In most tissues, these compounds reduce amino acid uptake and stimulate a pronounced catabolic action that induces a negative nitrogen balance leading to the atrophy of muscle, epidermal, and connective tissue. The amino acids derived from protein degradation are the substrate for the enhanced gluconeogenesis that concurrently occurs in the liver. The net effect is an increase in production of glucose-6-phosphate and in protein synthesis. The increase in glucose-6-phosphatase activity in the liver results in release of glucose into the blood and hyperglycemia, which stimulates diabetes (steroid diabetes) when glucocorticoids are in excess.

The effect of glucocorticoids on carbohydrate metabolism may be discussed in terms of acute and chronic phases (Figure 7.2). First, there is a rapid net transfer of amino acids from muscle to liver and kidney tissues, where preexisting gluconeogenic enzyme systems convert amino acids into glucose. There is also increased release of fatty acids and glycerol from adipose tissue to the liver, where the glycerol can contribute to glucogenesis and where the increased fatty acid level inhibits key liver glycolytic enzymes, thus reducing glucose breakdown. An increase in glycogen synthetase and pyruvic carboxylase activity contributes to an increase in liver glycogen. In the liver, glucocorticoids can induce the rapid biosynthesis of tyrosine transaminase, tryptophan oxygenase, orthinine decarboxylase, and glutamic-pyruvate transaminase. These gluconeogenic enzymes make the carbon skeletons of numerous amino acids available for subsequent glucogenesis. They show a familiar pattern of dependency on both RNA synthesis and the general protein synthetic machinery, since drugs which block these functions—for example, actinomycin D, cycloheximide, and puromycin—also prevent the glucocorticoid-stimulated increases of these enzymes as well as their gluconeogenic effects. This is a prime example of the involvement of a hormone in the transcriptional or translational machinery of the liver cell.

The most significant chronic effect of glucocorticoid action is the stimulation of biosynthesis of the enzymes involved in glucogenesis that divert carbohydrate precursors to glucose formation. These include four key enzymes as outlined in Figure 7.3: glucose-6-phosphatase, fructose diphosphatase, phosphoenolpyruvate car-

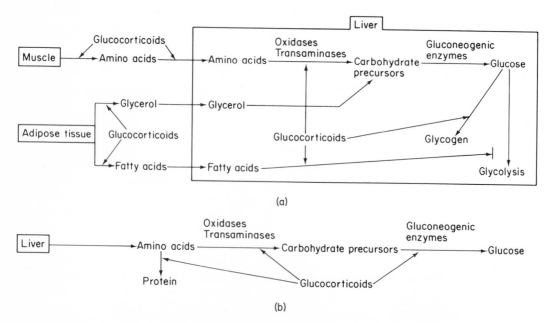

Figure 7.2 (a) Acute and (b) chronic effects of glucocorticoids on carbohydrate metabolism. The arrow ending in a bar (———▶│) indicates an inhibitory effect. Unblocked arrows indicate stimulation.

boxykinase, and pyruvate decarboxylase. These enzymes also appear to be affected at the level of protein biosynthesis much like the gluconeogenic enzymes. The interplay of the glucocorticoids and insulin in regulating the level of these enzymes is a remarkable illustration of hormone effects at the molecular and genetic level (Figure 7.3). It has been shown by Lardy and Weber and co-workers that in contrast to glucocorticoid stimulation, insulin acts as a suppressor of these glucogenic enzymes, inducing glycogenic and glycolytic enzymes. Weber has proposed that various groups of enzymes operate as functional genetic units, and that the antagonistic effects of glucocorticoids and insulin may operate at this basic level.

Virtually every feature of fat metabolism—oxidation, synthesis, mobilization, and storage—appears to be affected, probably indirectly, by the glucocorticoids. Cortisol induces transport of fat from subcutaneous tissues to the liver and serum; the resulting ketonuria and ketonemia indicate an increased rate of fatty acid oxidation. The steroid-induced lipogenesis is attributable to the increase in insulin secretion.

Other Effects of the Glucocorticoids

These hormones have a variety of significant physiological effects that apparently result indirectly from their glucocorticoid action. Many of these responses have been found to be most useful therapeutically. They include the remarkable anti-allergic and anti-inflammatory effects of the glucocorticoids. Lymphoid tissue (for example, thymus) and blood lymphocytes are decreased by adrenocortical secretions. Erythropoiesis is enhanced by glucocorticoid stimulation of bone mar-

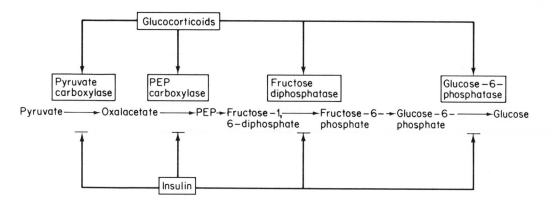

Figure 7.3   Antagonistic effects of glucocorticoids and insulin on liver glucogenic enzymes. In this and similar diagrams reflecting in vivo experiments, the arrows leading from the glucocorticoids to a particular enzyme are not meant to imply a direct effect on that enzyme. Likewise, the blocked arrows from insulin do not imply an inhibitory effect on the molecular mechanism of that particular enzyme. In fact, many of the effects of insulin can be produced by increasing the intracellular concentration of glucose. PEP is 2-phosphoenolpyruvate.

row metabolism. Finally, steroids with an oxy group at C-11 cause an augmentation of both hydrochloric acid and pepsinogen secretion by the gastric mucosa, as well as an increased output of pancreatic enzymes.

7.6 THE ADRENAL MEDULLA HORMONES

Epinephrine, the principal hormone of the adrenal medulla of most species, was the first hormone to be isolated and identified (by Abel in 1904). Since epinephrine is the primary product of the medulla, it is also the most prevalent form of the circulating hormone. Norepinephrine is present in smaller quantities in the adrenals but functions mainly as the neurotransmitter in the sympathetic nervous system and generally acts locally on effector cells. These two hormones, together with their precursor, dopamine, comprise a distinct group of substances; this group, the catecholamines, share a common *ortho*- dihydroxy structural feature. The catecholamines are the "emergency" hormones proposed by Walter Cannon over 50 yr ago, constituting the principal regulatory mechanism involved in the emergency reaction that permits the animal to mobilize to meet physical or emotional challenges.

The catecholamines are derived from tyrosine in a series of well-described biosynthetic steps shown in Figure 7.4. L-Tyrosine is specifically hydroxylated to form 3,4-dihydroxyphenylalanine (DOPA); tyrosine hydroxylase, the enzyme controlling this reaction, requires a tetrahydropteridine cofactor. This reaction is the rate-limiting regulatory step in the synthesis of epinephrine by the adrenals. Tyrosine hydroxylase is effectively inhibited in vivo by its analog, α-methyltyrosine, which

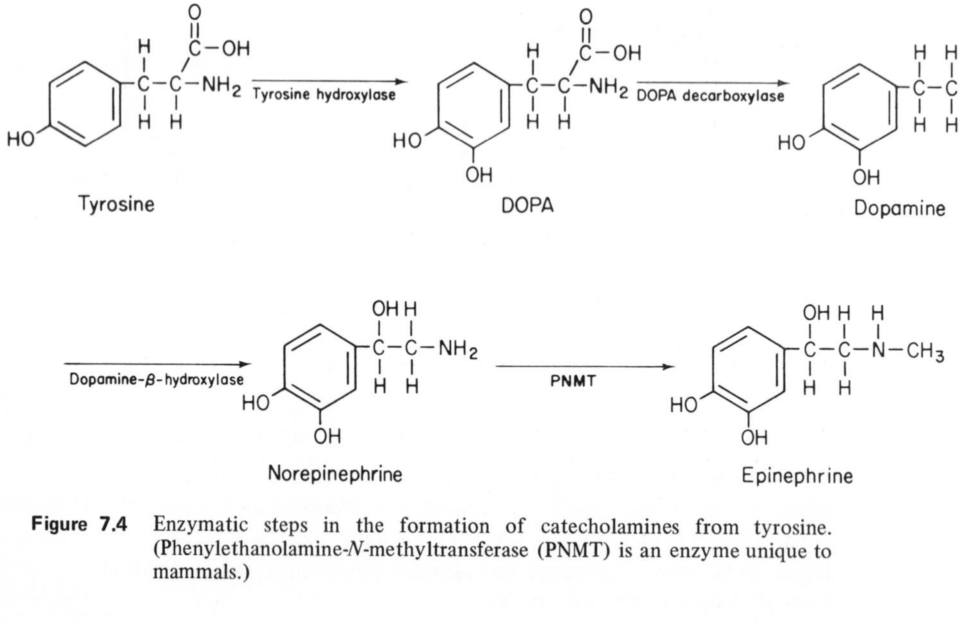

Figure 7.4 Enzymatic steps in the formation of catecholamines from tyrosine. (Phenylethanolamine-*N*-methyltransferase (PNMT) is an enzyme unique to mammals.)

can thus prevent the synthesis of epinephrine. Decarboxylation by DOPA decarboxylase is followed by a unique and specific hydroxylation, catalyzed by the copper enzyme dopamine-β-hydroxylase, also requiring ascorbic acid and oxygen. The adrenal medulla in the mammal has an additional enzyme, phenylethanolamine-N-methyltransferase; in combination with S-adenosyl methionine, this enzyme completes the methylation reaction and converts norepinephrine to epinephrine. The latter enzyme appears to be under the control of adrenocorticoids, since removal of the pituitary causes a significant decrease in the rate of the final epinephrine-forming step.

The simplicity of the catecholamine structure has led to extensive studies on the effect of structural variation on hormonal activity. However, the diversity of physiological effects (illustrated in Table 7.1) complicates the interpretation of these data. In general, the greatest sympathomimetic activity (mimicking the action of the sympathetic branch of the autonomic nervous system) occurs when two carbon atoms separate the benzene rings from the amino group. For maximal activity, the presence of the hydroxyl groups at C-3 and C-4 is required. The benzene ring is also essential for the stimulation of central-nervous system effects. Substitution of the a-carbon prolongs the duration of action of these compounds by decreasing the action of monoamineoxidase, which inactivates the catecholamines. Several phenylethylamine derivatives, for example, ephedrine and amphetamine, are clinically useful as sympathomimetic drugs because their effects are of longer duration than epinephrine or norepinephrine.

The metabolism of the catecholamines follow two principal but nonexclusive pathways, one leading to deamination by monoamineoxidase and the other involving O-methylation by catecholamine-O-methyltransferase. These two enzymes are not highly specific and account for the sequence of reactions shown in Figure 7.5, in which the initial reaction is either N-oxidation or catechol methylation. Most of the subsequent metabolites are rapidly excreted and thus are of limited importance.

7.7 CONTROL OF CATECHOLAMINE SECRETION

As in the cases of oxytocin and vasopressin, release of epinephrine is one of the few examples of direct neural control of hormone secretion (described in Figures 2.2, 2.16, and 2.17). Stimulation of the splanchnic nerve causes a secretion of these hormones; the cutting of this nerve or the direct application of nicotine greatly reduces their secretion. Cells of the adrenal medulla are derived embryologically from neural crest tissue; they are modified postganglionic cells that maintain contact with the preganglionic fibers of the sympathetic nervous system. Thus, secretory activity is largely regulated by the splanchnic nerves. Catecholamines are stored in cytoplasmic granules of the chromaffin cells and are discharged by nerve stimulation. These granules can reaccumulate the catecholamines or accumulate similar substances. Ephedrine and amphetamines also cause the discharge of the

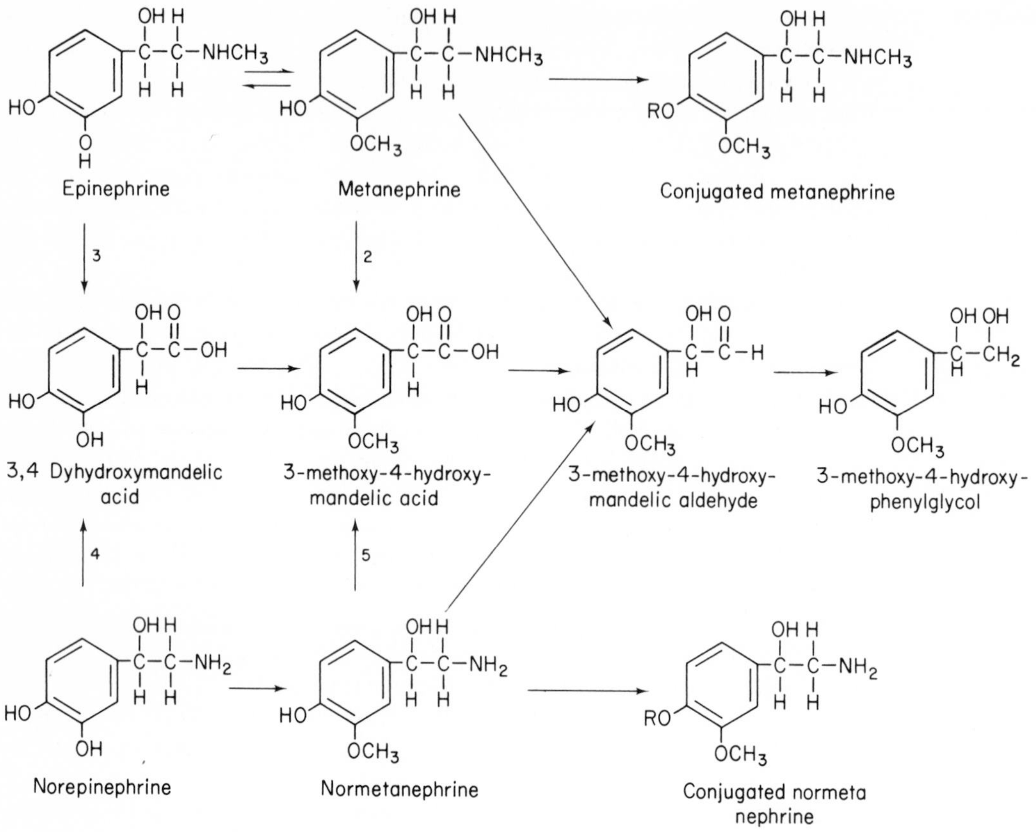

Figure 7.5   The metabolism of epinephrine and norepinephrine.

catecholamines from the granules, but at different rates. Recent data suggest that epinephrine and norepinephrine are formed by different cells of the medulla and may be released separately, depending upon the kind of stimulus.

7.8 METABOLIC EFFECTS OF EPINEPHRINE

A list of the numerous physiological effects of catecholamines is summarized in Table 7.1. Epinephrine exerts the principal metabolic effects. Its acute effects on carbohydrate metabolism are illustrated in Figure 7.6. As described by the Coris, there is a rapid increase both in blood sugar and lactate at the expense of liver glycogen, and later, of muscle glycogen. The hyperglycemic effect of epinephrine apparently arises not only from the activation of the phosphorylase system, but also from the inhibition of insulin secretion. Epinephrine also increases the free fatty acid level of the blood as much as 100 percent, apparently by promoting

TABLE 7.1 COMPARISON OF THE EFFECTS OF EPINEPHRINE
AND NOREPINEPHRINE IN MAN[a]

Response	Epinephrine	Norepinephrine
Metabolic		
Oxygen consumption	++	0,+
Blood sugar	+++	0,+
Blood lactic acid	+++	0,+
Eosinopenic response	+	0
Cardiac		
Heart rate	+	–
Stroke volume	++	++
Cardiac output	+++	0,–
Arrhythmias	++++	++++
Coronary blood flow	++	+++
Blood pressure		
Systolic arterial	+++	+++
Mean arterial	+	++
Diastolic arterial	+,0,–	++
Mean pulmonary	++	++
Peripheral circulation		
Total peripheral resistance	–	++
Cerebral blood flow	+	0,–
Muscle blood flow	++	0,–
Cutaneous blood flow	–,–	+,0,–
Renal blood flow	–	–
Splanchnic blood flow	++	0,+
Central Nervous System		
Respiration	+	+
Subjective sensations	+	0,+

[a] 0.1 to 0.4 μg/kg per min intravenous infusion; + = increase; 0 = no change; – = decrease. Modified from Goldenberg *et al, Archs. Intern. Med.,* **86**, 823, (1950).

lipolysis in adipose tissue. The increased availability of these oxidizable substrates, coupled with greater blood flow in muscle, results in a 20 to 30 percent elevation of oxygen consumption. The eosinopenic response, a decrease in eosinophil count, is believed to arise indirectly from an epinephrine-induced release of ACTH and a resulting increase in glucocorticoids; the latter also help to sustain the hyperglycemic response via gluconeogenesis. All of these responses fit into Cannon's "emergency" theory, in which epinephrine is assigned a central role in preparing the vertebrate to cope with a sudden environmental challenge.

7.9 CARDIOVASCULAR EFFECTS OF THE CATECHOLAMINES

The catecholamines cause widely differing responses in the smooth muscle of the cardiovascular system (see Table 7.1). Epinephrine causes a constriction of cutaneous arteriolar smooth muscle and a dilation (and consequent increase in blood

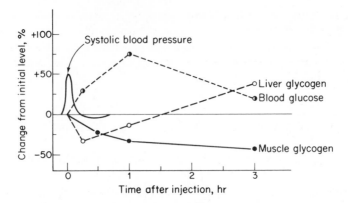

Figure 7.6 Effect of epinephrine (0.2 mg/kg body weight) on the blood glucose and tissue glycogen levels of the normal rat, as compared with the quick response of the cardiovascular system.

flow) through the blood vessels of the muscles in the limbs. The smooth muscles of the arterioles in the heart dilate, thus increasing the blood flow through the heart, but the arterioles of the abdominal viscera constrict. On isolated cardiac muscle, epinephrine increases the rate of contraction (chronotropic effect) and the strength of each contraction (inotropic effect). Its action on the intact heart is less clearly seen, but after the administration of epinephrine the heart rate slows and each heart beat is much stronger. These effects are secondary to reflexes induced by the increase in blood pressure and the initial increase in heart rate. This spectrum of responses has been explained by the assumption that there are two kinds of tissue target sites, α and β receptors. The blood vessels of the skin, mucosa, and kidney are constricted due to effects of epinephrine on their α receptors, whereas dilation of the vessels of the skeletal muscles is due to the hormone's action on their β receptors, which have a lower threshold to epinephrine than do the α receptors. Thus, low doses of epinephrine exclusively affect β receptors, lowering blood pressure; higher doses activate both receptors, resulting in an increase in peripheral resistance and a rise in blood pressure. As the epinephrine concentration falls below the threshold of the α receptor, the response of the β receptor predominates, producing a residual hypotension. The existence of two different kinds of receptors has also been used to account for differences in the responses to epinephrine and norepinephrine. For example, norepinephrine affects the α receptors, augmenting both systolic and diastolic blood pressure without affecting cardiac output.

Epinephrine produces a variety of effects on smooth muscle, both relaxing bronchial and gastrointestinal tract musculature and contracting the pyloric and ileocecal sphincters. None of these metabolic or muscular responses are induced by norepinephrine; however, the latter is the principal chemical mediator at the postganglionic adrenergic nerve endings.

While hypofunction of the adrenal medulla is unknown, hyperfunction can be induced by certain tumors (for example, chromaffin tissue tumors or pheo-chromocytomas). These tumors may increase the plasma level of epinephrine and norepinephrine 500 times and result in persistent hypertension. Elevation of the basal metabolic rate, hyperglycemia, and lipemia are all responses traceable to epinephrine action.

7.10 ACTION OF EPINEPHRINE IN RELATION TO CYCLIC AMP

The role of c-AMP as the second messenger was first discovered in 1960 by Suther-land and Rall when they attempted to account for the glycogenolytic effects of epinephrine in liver. As described in Chapter 4 (Figure 4.5), epinephrine, like glu-cagon, increases the rate of formation of c-AMP, which in turn increases the rate of formation of active glycogen phosphorylase, presumably by activating phosphory-lase kinase. Many of the other effects of epinephrine in liver, that is, stimulation of gluconeogenesis and production of gluconeogenic enzymes, involves c-AMP. In skeletal muscle, c-AMP levels increase in response to epinephrine. Additional evidence for the role of c-AMP is found in the facilitation of neuromuscular trans-mission effects of epinephrine by the action of theophylline, a phosphodiesterase inhibitor. Epinephrine also increases the c-AMP level in the perfused rabbit heart and rat smooth muscle. Sutherland and his associates have correlated a positive response to the adrenergic β receptors with the adenylcyclase system. These effects are reflected in the cardiovascular system as the positive inotropic, chronotropic, and vasodepressor effects of sympathetic stimulation, mediated by increases in the level of c-AMP at appropriate sites. The effects on a-receptor activation, resulting in vasoconstriction, may be related to a decrease in the intracellular level of c-AMP.

REFERENCES

Eisenstein, A. B. (ed.): *The Adrenal Cortex*, Little, Brown and Co., Boston, 1967.

von Euler, U. S.: "Chromaffin Cell Hormones," in U. S. von Euler and H. Heller (eds.), *Comparative Endocrinology*, vol. 1, Academic Press, Inc., New York, 1963.

Goodman, L. S., and A. Gilman: *The Pharmacological Basis of Therapeutics*, 3rd ed., The Macmillan Company, New York, 1967.

McKerns, K. W. (ed.): *Functions of the Adrenal Cortex*, vols. 1 and 2, Appleton-Century-Crofts, New York, 1968.

EIGHT | PARATHYROID HORMONE AND CALCITONIN

8.1 THE ROLE OF CALCIUM AND PHOSPHATE

Calcium exists in the plasma both in an ionized, dialyzable state and in a nonionized state largely bound to protein. The concentration of free Ca^{2+} is dependent upon the concentration of plasma proteins, as is indicated by the dissociation equilibrium determined by McLean and Hastings:

$$\frac{[Ca^{2+}] \times [Protein^{2-}]}{[Ca\text{-}protein]} = K = 10^{-2.2}$$

The concentration of free Ca^{2+} in the plasma at pH 7.35 is approximately half of the total concentration of Ca. The normal range of calcium in the plasma is between 4.5 and 5.5 milliequivalents (meq)/liter (90 to 110 mg/liter).

Calcium is biologically active only in the ionic state, participating in a number of processes. Calcium ions are intimately involved in the regulation of cellular activity

124

by controlling the irritability of cells. In the absence of adequate Ca^{2+}, nerves fire spontaneously, muscle cells show lowered threshold to stimuli, cardiac contractility is augmented, and relaxation is retarded. The increase in irritability associated with hypocalcemia, with characteristic clinical signs, is most frequently encountered in hypoparathyroidism, and is manifested as sustained and painful contractures of various sets of muscles. This phenomenon is known as tetany, and may be either latent (and triggered by a stimulus) or overt.

Lack of either adequate amounts of Ca^{2+} due to deficiency in the diet or adequate absorption due to vitamin-D deficiency results in formation of rachitic bones lacking in bone minerals. Calcium ions play a key role in blood coagulation. Collected blood does not coagulate if the Ca^{2+} is removed with oxalate or chelated with either citrate or ethylenediaminetetracetate (EDTA); clinically, however, such low concentrations of Ca^{2+} are not achieved in the bloodstream. Adhesion between cells is decreased and permeability of capillaries is increased when the Ca^{2+} concentration is sharply reduced. Muscle contraction is thought to be dependent on the release of traces of bound Ca by the nerve impulse so that the ionic form may activate the adenosine triphosphatase of myosin and cause splitting of ATP.

Phosphorus (as phosphate) is also an important element: it is present in the plasma in a concentration range of 1.4 to 2.9 meq/liter (25 to 50 mg/liter). The plasma phosphate concentration is inversely related to the concentration of Ca, that is, $[Ca] \times [PO_4] = K$. Phosphates are involved in a number of processes: they are part of the crystalline structure of the bone mineral hydroxyapatite, $Ca_{10}(PO_4)_6(OH)_2$; they form the backbone of nucleic acids; they are components of the nucleotides; and they are involved in membrane structures as phospholipids. Phosphorylation is an important mechanism in the intermediary metabolism of all foodstuffs. Phosphate compounds are also part of the buffer system of the plasma.

The renal nephron is capable of converting Na_2HPO_4 to NaH_2PO_4 as a means of conserving Na^+. The homeostasis of calcium and phosphates is primarily based on the interaction in the target tissues of two hormones, parathyroid hormone (PTH) and calcitonin (CT).

8.2 ANATOMY AND CHEMISTRY

The parathyroid glands have the distinction of being among the last of the vertebrate glands to be discovered. They were described initially by Owen more than 100 years ago and again by Sandstrom in 1880, but the reports went unnoticed until the glands were rediscovered by Gley in 1891. The glands develop as two pairs of small, yellowish bodies on the surface of the thyroid gland, but on occasion they may be embedded in the thyroid tissue. The variable effects obtained when the parathyroids are removed are due to the presence of accessory glands in the thorax. The parathyroids are composed of two types of cells, a relatively small *principal cell* (or chief cell), and the *oxyphil cell*, characterized by its purple staining granules. The chief cell is the source of PTH, the hypercalcemic hormone. The bovine hormone is a single polypeptide chain with a molecular weight of 9,500. It is composed of 83 amino acid residues and contains 17 of the common amino acids but lacks cysteine. A tentative structure proposed by Potts is shown in Figure 8.1. Oxidation of methionine, tyrosine, or tryptophan causes complete loss of biological activity, as does acetylation or esterification. Removal of the last four amino acids from the C-terminal portion by digestion with carboxypeptidase has no effect on activity, but removal of the next four to five amino acids causes marked loss of activity. Weak acid hydrolysis ruptures the peptide bonds of aspartic acid, yielding free aspartic acid and several polypeptide fragments. The largest fragment contains 20 amino acid residues and when purified shows biological and immunological activity. This fragment retains activity after carboxypeptidase digestion, although it is reduced to 16 amino acids. Further reduction in length by treatment with cyanogen bromide, causing cleavage at methionine, still does not destroy immunological activity.

Extracts of ultimobranchial glands of chickens, turkeys, chum salmon, and grey cod contain a factor that induces hypocalcemia in young rats. Copp has therefore sugested that his original term for the hypocalcemic factor, calcitonin, is more appropriate than thyrocalcitonin, the term introduced by Hirsch when he found the hypocalcemic factor in thyroid gland extracts.

The ultimobranchial gland in jawed vertebrates arises from the last branchial pouch. However, in amphibians the parathyroids develop from the third and fourth branchial pouches, suggesting that the organs controlling Ca metabolism are derived from the branchial pouches. In mammals, the ultimobranchial glands are no longer discrete but are incorporated into the thyroid gland as dispersed cells. The upper pole of the rabbit thyroid gland has no parafollicular cells and extracts lack hypocalcemic activity. Bovine CT, with a molecular weight of 3,600, contains 32 amino acids, including two half-cystines and one methionine. In 1968, three pharmaceutical research groups announced the total synthesis of CT. The amino acid sequence for synthetic porcine CT is shown in Figure 8.2.

8.3 REGULATION OF SECRETION

The most generally accepted hypothesis to explain Ca homeostasis is that suggested by McLean and Urist. They proposed that the Ca^{2+} concentration in the plasma acts through negative feedback to regulate the secretion of PTH. The stimulus for increased PTH secretion is a decline in the plasma Ca^{2+} concentration by 0.4 mg to 1.0 mg/100 ml. The McLean-Urist hypothesis has been expanded to include the role of CT (Figure 8.3). Elevation of Ca^{2+} from 0.15 mg to 0.5 mg/100 ml plasma is sufficient to provoke a secretion of CT causing a decline in the plasma Ca^{2+} concentration. The action of CT is quickly apparent and persists for only a brief time, whereas that of PTH occurs more slowly and persists much longer. These hormones

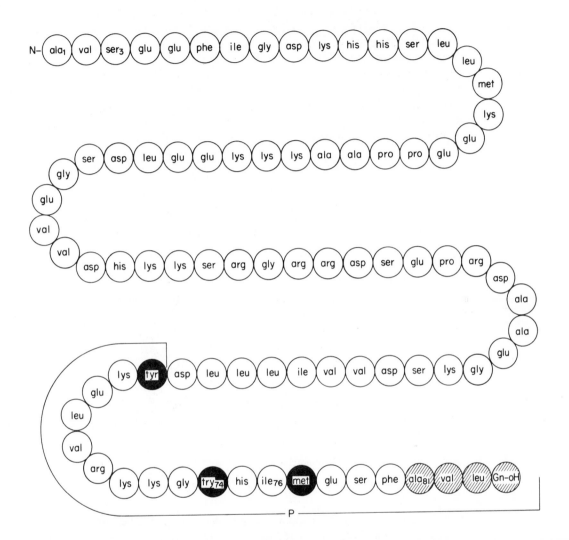

Figure 8.1 Tentative amino acid sequence of the parathyroid hormone molecule illustrating regions important for biological and immunological activity. The cross-hatched residues at the COOH-terminus were not necessary for biological activity but alteration of methionine, trypotophan, and tyrosine residues (shown by symbols with darkened borders) caused marked loss of biological activity. The 20-amino acid region (HP$_3$) at the carboxylterminus is a biologically and immunologically active fragment. [Modified from J. T. Potts, Jr. G. D. Aurbach, and L. M. Sherwood, "Parathyroid Hormone: Chemical Properties and Structural Requirements for Biological and Immunological Activity," *Recent Progr. Hormone Res.*, **22**, 101 (1966).]

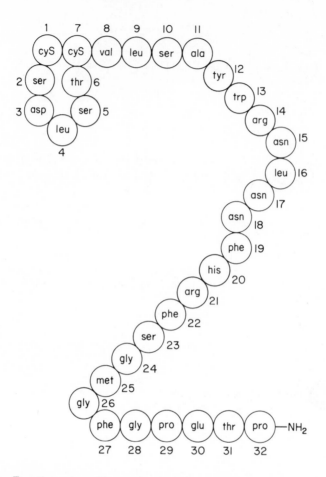

Figure 8.2 Tentative amino acid sequence of porcine calcitonin.

effectively regulate plasma calcium and phosphate concentrations over a narrow range of variation. Copp has chosen to refer to this control as a "push-pull" feedback system.

Talmage has shown that calcium and phosphate dissolve out of living or dead bone into plasma previously depleted of these substances. He also found that living or dead bone becomes a depository for calcium and phosphate when it is incubated with normal plasma. It is apparent that bone is in chemical equilibrium with calcium and phosphate ions of the plasma, and that the bones need not be living tissue. The bone salts that are in chemical equilibrium with the plasma are readily mobilizable; they are not the deeply buried bone salts whose release requires the activation of bone cells. The plasma calcium and phosphate-regulating hormones act on the bone cells. This effect is slow, however, compared to the rapid effect on the kidney.

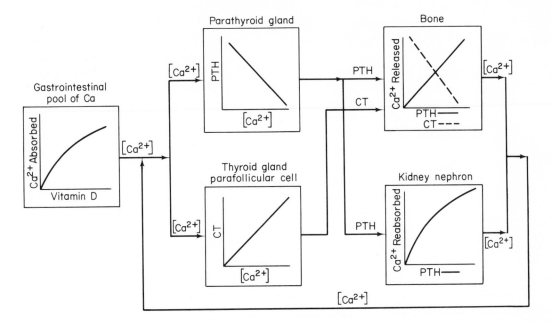

Figure 8.3   Control of $[Ca^{2+}]$ homeostasis by the negative feedback of the $[Ca^{2+}]$ on the parathyroid gland, causing the secretion of parathyroid hormone (PTH), and on the parafollicular cell, regulating the secretion of calcitonin (CT).

8.4   EFFECT OF PARATHYROID AND CALCITONIN

PTH acts on the osteoclasts of bone to promote dissolution of bone minerals. This effect is seen both in PTH implants near bone in vivo and in the accelerated release of radioactive calcium (^{45}Ca) from labeled fetal bone when grown in vitro. The mechanism by which Ca is actively released from bone is not clear. Suggested ideas include: (1) disruption of the collagen strands by collagenase, releasing bone minerals for rapid solution; (2) dissolution of bone minerals by excess formation of citrates or lactates; and (3) a change in permeability characteristics of cells so that Ca transport proceeds from bone to body fluids. In part, these ideas are based on the association of increased reabsorption of osteocollagenous fibers with increased excretion of hydroxyproline.

The action of PTH on the kidney is seen in the decreased amount of Ca salts appearing in the urine. The action of PTH on the intestinal mucosa is not as clear-cut; however, the consensus is that Ca absorption is facilitated after the hormone is administered. After the administration of actinomycin D to rats, PTH fails to induce a hypercalcemia or a phosphaturia, indicating that biosynthetic reactions precede the expression of the hormonal effect on bone.

Calcitonin causes a prompt hypocalcemia and hypophosphatemia of short duration. Until purified samples of the hormone are available in larger amounts, measurements of its activity must be based on a biological assay and expressed in units. The Medical Research Council (Great Britain) has available for distribution a preparation called *Research Standard B for Thyroid Calcitonin,* which allows all workers to express the activity of their preparations in similar units. The MRC unit is the activity contained in one ampule. The biological response to 10 MRC milliunits is the reduction of blood Ca by approximately 10 percent in starved 150-g rats 1 hr after intravenous administration. The MRC unit is equivalent to 100 Hirsch units. Hirsch has defined one unit as the amount of hormone that depresses the serum Ca concentration of rats by 1 mg/100 ml. A dose of 5 to 10 Hirsch units produces a decrease in the serum Ca concentration to 7 to 8 mg/100 ml in 1 hr with a return to control values (about 10 mg/100 ml serum) in 1 to 3 hr more. The short duration of the CT effect is due to activation of PTH secretion. In the parathyroidectomized rat, the action of CT persists for many hours. It increases the uptake of Ca by bone cells (osteoblasts). The action of PTH on the osteoclasts of bone is apparently blocked by CT since the PTH-induced discharge of ^{45}Ca from prelabeled bone ceases when CT is added to the medium. Calcitonin has no effect on renal excretion of phosphate except in large doses, when it causes a hypophosphatemia and hyperphosphaturia; at low doses a hyperphosphaturia is due to increased secretion of parathyroid hormone. It is probable that no new protein biosynthesis is involved in CT-induced hypocalcemia, as actinomycin D has no effect.

8.5 OTHER CONTROLS ON CALCIUM METABOLISM

Calcium metabolism is also influenced by vitamin D, which regulates the synthesis of a Ca-binding protein in the mucosa of the gastrointestinal tract. A calcium-binding protein may be necessary for the absorption of Ca from the intestine. Growth of long bone under the influence of GH results in an increased amount of organic matrix on which Ca may accumulate and on which bone minerals may condense under the influence of osteoblasts. Estrogens cause an arrest of bone growth by causing closure of the growing ends (the epiphyses) of the long bones, and they exert a stabilizing action on Ca metabolism. This effect becomes apparent in menopausal women; with cessation of ovarian function, they show a concomitant, increased resorption of bone mineral with a consequent rarification.

Thyroid hormones also play a significant role in the metabolism of Ca and the regulation of bone maturation. The action of GH on bone growth is enhanced in the presence of thyroid hormone. In the absence of thyroid hormones, the epiphyses fail to grow normally and ossification is disturbed. In hyperthyroid animals there is an increased excretion of Ca in the urine and feces, and the blood Ca may vary from a normal to a hypercalcemic concentration. In long-standing thyroid-hormone deficiency, bone rarefaction is seen. Clinically, hyperparathyroidism manifests itself by resorption of bone minerals, and in extreme conditions, by deforma-

TABLE 8.1 SUBSTANCES THAT AFFECT CALCIUM METABOLISM

Substance	Source	Chemical Nature	Site of Action	Effect
Vitamin D	Diet	Steroid	Intestinal mucosa	Increases Ca^{2+}-binding protein, facilitating absorption of Ca^{2+}
Calcitonin (hypocalcamic factor)	Thyroid (ultimobranchial gland)	Polypeptide MW = 3,500–4,000	Bone (increases deposition of calcium salts)	Decreases serum Ca^{2+}, Mg^{2+}, urinary hydroxy-proline, and PO_4^{3-}
Parathyroid hormone (hypercalcemic factor)	Parathyroid	Polypeptide MW = 8,447	Bone (activates osteoclastic cells, causing resorption of bone)	Increases serum Ca^{2+}, Mg^{2+} and urinary PO_4^{3-} and hydroxproline
			Kidney (increases reabsorption of Ca^{2+})	
			Intestinal mucosa (synergizes vitamin D action)	
Growth hormone	Adenohypophysis	Polypeptide	Bone (activates osteoblasts)	Increases utilization of Ca^{2+} during growth
Estradiol	Ovary (adrenal cortex)	Steroid	Bone (activates osteoblasts)	Causes closure of epiphyses, prevents resorption of Ca^{2+}
Thyroid hormones	Thyroid	Iodo amino acids	Bone (activates osteoblasts)	In growing animal, exerts permissive effect for growth hormone necessary for maturation of ends of bone; in adults, prevents resorption of Ca^{2+}

tion of bone. The condition of postparturent paresis in cows may be due to excessive secretion of CT, as this hormone is associated with a hypocalcemia and hypophosphaturia. Table 8.1 summarizes the substances exerting an influence on Ca metabolism.

REFERENCES

McLean, F. C., and M. R. Urist: *Bone*, University of Chicago Press, Chicago, 1961.

Potts, J. T., Jr., G. D. Aurbach, and L. M. Sherwood: "Parathyroid Hormone: Chemical Properties and Structural Requirements for Biological and Immunological Activity," *Recent Progr. Hormone Res.*, **22**, 101-142 (1966).

Talmage, R. V., and others: A Symposium on Comparative Aspects of Parathyroid Function. *Amer. Zool.*, **7**, 823-895 (1967).

Talmage, R. V. (ed.): *Parathyroid Glands and Thyrocalcitonin (Calcitonin)*, Excerpt Medica Foundation, Amsterdam, 1968.

NINE | OTHER VERTEBRATE HORMONES

Numerous substances with hormonal properties have been and continue to be described. Generally, these are discovered by injection of crude organ extracts into test animals, by applying extracts to smooth muscle strips, or by other suitable test systems. In the study of endocrinology, the role of these substances is uncertain until the criteria already described in Chapter 1 can be satisfied. Because of our arbitrary definition of hormones, we have tentatively excluded as bona fide hormones such substances as serotonin, prostaglandin, histamine, and the kinins. These are indeed highly active substances affecting many tissues but their actions are local and not dependent on their transport in the blood or lymph. At this time, we have no way of distinguishing between these substances and other highly active and functional metabolites. Therefore, such substances are excluded from the roster of miscellaneous hormones discussed in this chapter.

9.1 THE GASTROINTESTINAL HORMONES

A number of substances have been extracted from the mucosa of the gastrointestinal tract (Figure 9.1) that affect either secretory or motor activity of other parts of the tract and can exert this effect when injected intravenously. These hormones are polypeptides; the amino acid sequences of two of these substances have been determined (Figure 9.2). Gastrin, a heptadecapeptide, is structurally different for each of the species in which it has been studied except for cows and sheep. It causes an increase in the secretion of acid-containing gastric juice. A controversy still exists over whether gastrin acts directly on the stomach parietal cell or causes the release of histamine, which stimulates the partietal cells. Hist-

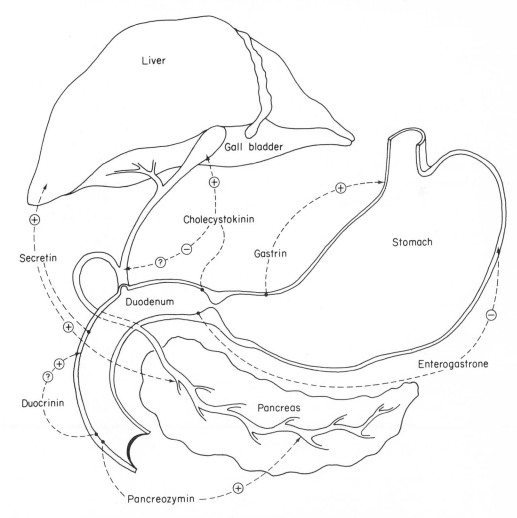

Figure 9.1   Diagram showing the origin and action of six gastro-intestinal hormones. The place of origin and site of action of each of these six hormones are entirely within the digestive tract, but they are carried from one place to another by the systemic circulation. A stimulatory action is indicated by a plus sign; an inhibitory action is indicated by a minus sign. (Modified from A. Gorbman and H. A. Bern, *A Textbook of Comparative Endocrinology,* Wiley, New York, 1962, p. 194.)

Gastrin

```
         1     2     3     4     5     6     7     8     9    10    11    12    13    14    15    16    17
Human: gly - gly - pro - try - leu - glu - glu - glu - glu - glu - ala - tyr - gly - try - met - asp - phe - NH2
                                                                            |
                                                                            R
                       5
Pig:                 -met-

                       5     6     7     8     9    10
Dog:                 -met - glu - ala - glu - glu -

                       5     6     7     8     9    10
Cow and sheep:       -val - glu - glu - glu - ala -
```

Secretin

```
       1     2     3     4     5     6     7     8     9    10    11    12    13    14    15    16    17    18    19    20    21    22    23    24    25    26    27
Pig: his - ser - asp - gly - thr - phe - thr - ser - glu - leu - ser - arg - leu - arg - asp - ser - ala - arg - leu - gln - arg - leu - leu - gln - gly - leu - val - NH2
```

Figure 9.2 Amino acid sequence of several gastrins and pig secretin. Except where indicated, amino acid sequences are identical to human gastrin. R on position 12 of gastrin is –H or -SO$_3$H. [The sequences are derived from V. Mutt and J. E. Jorpes, "Contemporary Developments in the Biochemistry of the Gastrointestinal Hormones," *Recent Progr. Hormone Res.*, **23**, 483 (1967).]

amine by itself is able to emulate the effects of gastrin. Almost all of the biological activity of gastrin is found in the C-terminal tetrapeptide, try-met-asp-phe-NH$_2$. A change of the aspartic acid residue of this tetrapeptide causes loss of activity, whereas an alteration of the other amino acids has no effect on activity.

Secretin, first described by Starling and Bayliss in 1902, was finally isolated in 1959, identified in 1965, and synthesized in 1966. It is a polypeptide composed of 27 amino acids (Figure 9.2). The sequence of the first 14 amino acids on the N-terminal end is similar but not identical to that of glucagon. Since secretin is a strongly basic molecule, it is firmly bound to cell proteins at the pH of body fluids; it is released into the blood or extracted from the antral duodenal mucosa by strong acids. Secretin causes the flow of a watery pancreatic juice that is high in salt content but low in enzymes.

Ivy described cholecystokinin, an intestinal mucosa extract that causes the gall bladder to contract, and Harper and Roper described pancreozymin, an intestinal mucosa extract that causes the pancreas to secrete a juice high in enzyme content. Mutt and Jorpes have isolated a tritriacontapeptide (33 amino acid residues), which they have called cholecystokinin-pancreozymin; it has the properties of the two hormones described earlier. This molecule has been cleaved by thrombin into an N-terminal inactive hexapeptide and a C-terminal active heptacosapeptide (27 amino acid residues). A C-terminal octapeptide, asp-try-(SO$_3$H)-met-gly-try-met-asp-phe-NH$_2$, retains much of the activity of the parent molecule. The C-terminal pentapeptide is identical to that of gastrin, indicating a possible relationship in the biosyntheses of these two intestinal hormones.

A number of other gastrointestinal hormones have been investigated, but little is known of their chemistry. These include the following: enterocrinin, controlling the secretion of intestinal juice; villikinin, controlling the movement of the villi; and duocrinin, controlling the secretion from Brunner's glands, which are located in the submucosa of the upper duodenum.

Enterogastrone exerts a negative effect by inhibiting gastric motility and secretion. It was first described by Ewald and Boas in 1886, but its chemical nature has not yet been determined. It is secreted by the mucosa of the duodenum and jejunum into the blood when high concentrations of fat, fatty digestion products, or carbohydrates are ingested. The evidence for its existence is based in part on the inhibition of motility and by secretion in an isolated stomach pouch, occurring after a fatty meal. The active factor can be extracted from duodenal musoca after the mucosa is first exposed to olive oil, whereas extracts from mucosa not exposed to lipids are inactive. Enterogastrone inhibits gastric activity arising from stimulation of the antrum of the stomach but only minimally inhibits gastric effects resulting from histamine stimulation.

9.2 RENAL HORMONES

The kidney is the source of two proteins: (1) the enzyme renin; and (2) erythropoietin, which may also function as an enzyme. These proteins exert widely different effects, but both generate hormonal activity by the proteolytic modification of a specific plasma-precursor protein.

Renin-Angiotensin

The presence of a pressor substance in kidney extracts has been known for 70 yr. The circulatory role of this hormone was established by Goldblatt *et al.* in 1934, when he and his associates produced persistent hypertension by constricting the renal arteries. The kidney factor renin was later found to be dependent on a serum protein for its hypertensive activity. The details of the process, shown in Figure 9.3, now have been determined by Page, Braun-Menendez, and co-workers. Renin acts as a specific protease, cleaving a decapeptide, angiotensin I, from the α_2-globulin, angiotensinogen. It remains for a specific peptidase or converting enzyme of the serum to convert the inactive angiotensin I to angiotensin II by removing two C-terminal amino acids, leu and his.

The control of the renin-angiotensin system has been described earlier in Chapter 7 and in Figure 7.1. The output of renin is reduced by an increase in renal blood pressure and by elevated plasma Na^+ and angiotensin II levels.

Effect of Angiotensin II

Though renin is the specific hormone secreted by the kidney, its ultimate biological effect is exerted by angiotensin II. The latter is the most powerful hypertensive agent known, having 40 times the activity of norepinephrine. A dose of

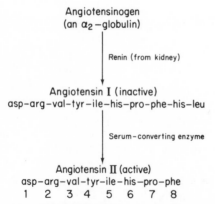

Angiotensinogen
(an α_2 −globulin)

Renin (from kidney)

Angiotensin I (inactive)
asp−arg−val−tyr−ile−his−pro−phe−his−leu

Serum−converting enzyme

Angiotensin II (active)
asp−arg−val−tyr−ile−his−pro−phe
1   2   3   4   5   6   7   8

Figure 9.3   The composition and sequence of the formation of angiotensins. The angiotensins shown are those isolated from horse serum. Ox angiotensins have valine rather than isoleucine in position 5. This slight variation in amino acid composition has no significant effect on pharmacological activity and is similar to the species variation in antidiuretic hormone composition.

0.002 μg/kg per minute will increase systemic blood pressure. Continuous infusion of angiotensin II has maintained an elevated blood pressure for hours or days. No inhibiting agent will interfere with the action of this octapeptide in vivo. In vitro, it constricts perfused vascular beds and contracts arterial strips, clearly establishing that it has a direct stimulant action on vascular smooth muscle, particularly in the vessels of the kidney, skin, and splanchnic region. In fact, the renal blood vessels are so sensitive to the vasoconstrictor action of angiotensin II that low doses effectively reduce both renal blood flow and glomerular filtration. This leads to a decreased excretion of both water and electrolyte in many species. In rodents and dogs, a transient antidiuresis is followed by a profuse diuresis, due to the inhibition of sodium reabsorption in the distal tubule by angiotensin II. This peptide exerts a third, indirect effect on kidney function by increasing aldosterone secretion by the adrenal cortex; this leads in turn to an antinatriuretic effect (increased Na^+ reabsorption).

Erythropoietin

People living at high altitudes for prolonged periods respond to this environmental stress with an increase in the number of circulating erythrocytes (erythrocytosis). As a result, it was mistakenly believed that the low pO_2 (partial pressure of oxygen) in the bone marrow was the stimulus. In 1906, Carnot and Deflandre demonstrated that an acute anemia (induced by hemorrhage) caused the appearance in the plasma of a factor capable of stimulating bone marrow in normal animals. Through the ingenious use of parabiotic rats with one parabiont maintained in a hypoxic environment, Reissman showed in 1950 that the bone marrow of the parabiont at normal pO_2 was also stimulated. Erslev then showed in 1953 that large volumes of plasma from anemic rabbits contained a factor that caused an erythropoiesis. In 1957, Jacobsen *et al.* showed that the kidneys were a probable source of the circulating factor, which by this time was generally referred to as erythropoietin. An increased production of erythropoietin can be caused either by anemia (due to hemorrhage or any factors that cause increased destruction of erythrocytes) or by the action of cobaltous salts upon the kidney. Erythropoietin induces hyperplasia of the bone marrow and an increase in the numbers of circulating reticulocytes, possibly by stimulating differentiation of multipotential stem cells into erythrocyte-precursor cells. The differentiated cells also show an enhanced rate of hemoglobin synthesis.

Erythropoietin is contained in the boiled and acidified fluid fraction of plasma. It has been identified as a glycoprotein with a molecular weight of 50,000 to 60,000. It contains about 30 percent carbohydrate, consisting of equal amounts of hexosamine and sialic acid. Since neuraminidase inactivates erythropoietin, the sialic acid moiety is necessary for biological activity.

The light mitochondrial fraction of rat kidneys contains an erythropoietic factor, the amount of which can be increased by prior treatment of the rats with a hypoxic environment [0.42 atmospheres (atm) for 19 hr] or with cobaltous ions. The supernatant of the light mitochondrial fraction is inactive in test animals unless it is previously incubated with serum. The concentration of erythropoietic activity increases if the serum was previously treated with ethylenediaminetetraacetate, dialyzed, and supplemented with $CaCl_2$. Although these observations are preliminary, Gordon's group has drawn the obvious parallel to the renin-angiotensin system.

9.3 THE PINEAL GLAND

The pineal gland was known to the early anatomists and in the seventeenth century was designated the "seat of the soul" by Descarates. The gland is located between the cerebral hemispheres, deep in the brain of most mammals. It is a vestige of the primitive, light-sensitive structure of lower vertebrates. In 1958, Lerner isolated and identified melatonin, a serotonin derivative from pineal gland tissue that causes bleaching in frog skin. Subsequently, Axelrod showed that pineal gland tissue was unique in possessing the enzyme hydroxyindole-O-methyl transferase, the enzyme that caused methylation of the hydroxyl group of n-acetyl serotonin, forming melatonin (Figure 9.4).

Constant exposure of a rat to light causes the ovaries to enlarge and the pineal glands to shrink. Pinealectomy causes the ovaries and the testes of rats to enlarge; however, the increase in gonad size following pinealectomy is blocked by administration of melatonin. Melatonin given daily in small amounts beginning before puberty causes the ovaries to be smaller than normal.

Synthesis of melatonin in the pineal gland is regulated by the amount of light to which the animal is exposed. Continuous light decreases the activity of the rate-limiting enzyme hydroxyindole-O-methyl transferase by a factor of 5 in rat pineal glands. Blinding hamsters causes the enzyme activity to double.

Melatonin inserted into the median eminence or reticular formation of the brain causes reduction in the pituitary LH content; continuous light causes increased secretion of LRH and LH production by the pituitary. The alternation of light and dark may control pineal gland secretion of melatonin and the latter may regulate the release of the hypothalamic gonadotrophin-releasing hormones (LRH and FRH) and ultimately regulate secretion of the pituitary gonadotrophins.

9.4 THE THYMUS

According to Sir M. Burnet, several endocrine factors are associated with the thymus in the mammal. There may be at least three thymic hormones, all responsible for primary lymphopoiesis. The best known thymus factor is necessary for the successful colonization of secondary lymphoidal organs by immunocytes from the thymus. A second factor regulates lymphopoiesis in the bursa-like organs. Both of these factors are secreted by thymic epithelial-reticular cells. A third substance is needed for the development of immunocytes into plasma cells capable of

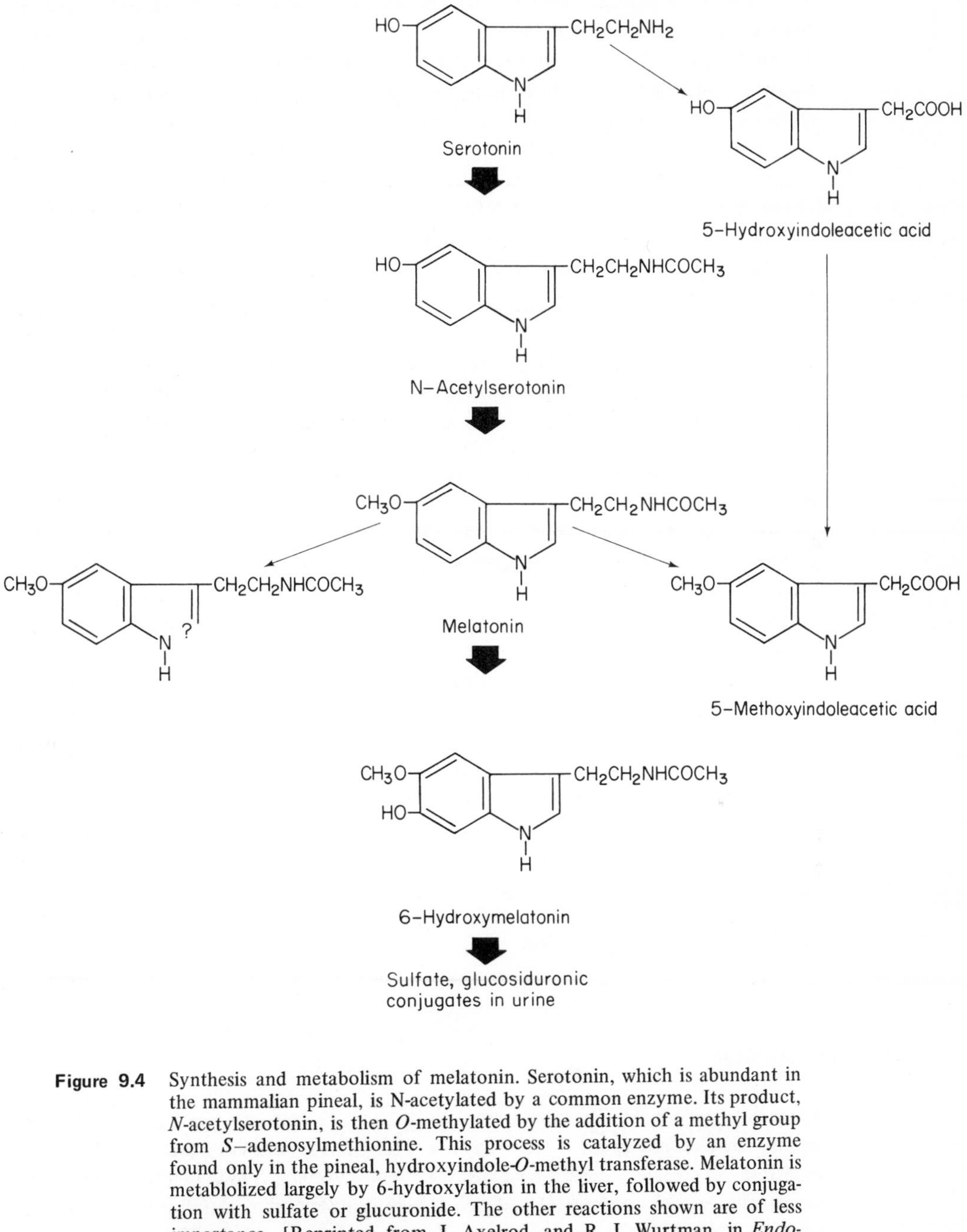

Figure 9.4 Synthesis and metabolism of melatonin. Serotonin, which is abundant in the mammalian pineal, is N-acetylated by a common enzyme. Its product, *N*-acetylserotonin, is then *O*-methylated by the addition of a methyl group from *S*–adenosylmethionine. This process is catalyzed by an enzyme found only in the pineal, hydroxyindole-*O*-methyl transferase. Melatonin is metabolized largely by 6-hydroxylation in the liver, followed by conjugation with sulfate or glucuronide. The other reactions shown are of less importance. [Reprinted from J. Axelrod, and R. J. Wurtman, in *Endocrines and the Central Nervous System* (Proceedings of the Association for Research in Nervous and Mental Disease), p. 200, The Williams & Wilkins Co., Baltimore, 1966.]

synthesizing immunoglobulins. It is produced by gut-associated epithelial-lymphoid organs.

Thymectomy results in a reduced lymphocyte population and loss of immunological competence; this is most pronounced in young animals. Regeneration of lymphocytes is greatly retarded in X-irradiated animals thymectomized prior to exposure to radiation. Appropriate thymic extracts, rich in soluble protein, will restore the growth of lymphoid tissue. Certain concentrated extracts, one of which has been named thymosin by White *et al.*, cause a hypertrophy of lymphoid tissue. Purification of thymus extracts has yielded an active glycopeptide, having a molecular weight of about 3,000.

REFERENCES

Axelrod, J., and R. J. Wurtman: "The Formation, Metabolism, and Some Actions of Melatonin, a Pineal Gland Substance," in *Endocrine and the Central Nervous System* (Proceedings of the Association for Research in Nervous and Mental Diseases), The William & Wilkins Co., Baltimore, 1966.

Fisher, J. W.: *Ann. N.Y. Acad. Sci.,* **149**, 1-583 (1968).

Page, I. H., and F. M. Bumpus: "Angiotensin," *Physiol. Rev.,* **41**, 331-390 (1961).

Recent Progr. in Hormone Res., **23** (1967). (A current summary of gastrointestinal, thymus, and other hormones.)

TEN

INTEGRATION AND MECHANISMS OF HORMONE ACTION

10.1 INTEGRATION OF THE PRIMARY EFFECTS OF HORMONES ON METABOLISM

Evolution of higher vertebrates has been accompanied by the development of an intricate set of hormonal controls that regulate cell processes. The continuous activity of the endocrine glands provides a chronic level of regulation, whereas the ability of the glands to secrete larger amounts of hormones as needed allows for acute regulation. The combination of chronic and acute regulation at the multicellular level contributes to the integrated behavior of organ systems, resulting in the delicate balance known as homeostasis. At virtually all levels of cellular organization, these controls influence the direction and route of metabolism, affecting the rate of transport by altering permeability of cell membranes, and altering nucleic acid and protein synthesis as well as the overall metabolism of carbohydrates, fats, and proteins. In this last chapter, an overall view of hormonal influences on the chemical machinery of the cell is presented. Figure 10.1 summarizes some of the numerous endocrine effects.

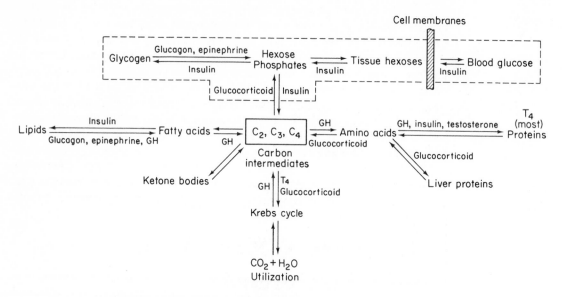

Figure 10.1 Overall effects of hormones in regulating the utilization of the principal metabolic classes. The area enclosed in the dashed lines indicates the acute control of carbohydrate metabolism in relation to blood glucose. The identification of a hormone action indicates positive in vivo effects on the metabolic sequence in the direction of the arrow.

Regulation of Carbohydrate Metabolism

A starting point for integrating and correlating the acute effects of hormones on carbohydrate metabolism is illustrated by the rapid control of blood sugar concentrations. The blood sugar concentration in the postabsorptive state is an indicator of the overall balance of carbohydrate metabolism; it reflects the equilibrium between the release of glucose from the liver and the demands of metabolism by the other tissues under the influence of intracellular and hormonal controls. The key steps in glucose homeostasis are diagrammed in the dashed area in Figure 10.1. The rapid hyperglycemic effects of glucagon and epinephrine on blood sugar are balanced by the increased secretion of the hypoglycemic hormone, insulin. In the normal animal with adequate supplies of carbohydrate as a precursor, these hormones play a major role in the minute-by-minute control of blood glucose concentration. Glucagon and epinephrine freely tap liver glycogen, which serves as a reservoir of glucose by stimulating the adenycyclase mechanism involved in glycogenolysis. The hypoglycemic effect of insulin is manifested at numerous key metabolic junctures; it includes greater glycogenesis and sugar uptake by many tissues as well as longer term effects on reduced gluconeogenesis.

The chronic effects of hormones on carbohydrate metabolism are manifested on blood glucose indirectly but significantly. Three additional major hormonal influences are involved in causing hyperglycemia, though the initiating factors may vary widely. The glucocorticoid stimulation of gluconeogenesis and glucogenesis, the greater rate of glycogenolysis and other metabolic reactions promoted by thyroid hormones, and the inhibition of glucose utilization by GH all tend to produce a hyperglycemia which must be balanced by insulin. Insulin not only moves glucose from the blood to the tissues for greater utilization but also promotes the formation of fat from carbohydrate precursors. The antagonistic effects of insulin and the glucocorticoids on gluconeogenesis and carbohydrate utilization were indicated in Chapters 4 and 7 and the diabetogenic action of GH and thyroid hormones was also previously noted.

The important effects of GH, glucocorticoids, insulin, and the thyroid hormones in promoting selected aspects of protein synthesis by stimulating the conversion of amino acids to certain proteins are qualitatively quite significant; however, they do not shift carbohydrate metabolism to a noncatabolic direction.

Regulation of Lipid Metabolism

Hormone action exerts significant effects on lipid metabolism through the control of lipolysis and the release of fatty acids from lipid stores. The fatty acid content of the blood in turn seems to regulate the rate of lipid oxidation by the tissues. Several hormones—epinephrine, glucagon, and GH—stimulate lipid breakdown and utilization by activating lipases which catalyze the hydrolysis of triglycerides to release fatty acids. The action of these hormones on lipase may involve c-AMP as an intermediate chemical signal. The augmentation of fat oxidation resulting from epinephrine and glucagon action represents a potential adaptive response, since fat can then be used as an auxiliary source of energy, conserving or supplementing glucose.

The primary balance in conserving triglycerides is provided by insulin. In promoting glucose uptake by adipose tissue, insulin increases the supply and utilization of carbohydrate, sparing C_2 units so that these can be diverted to the synthesis of triglycerides and cholesterol. The insulin effect in regulating this inverse relation between glucose and lipid metabolism is dependent on adequate dietary carbohydrate. In the absence of insulin or glucose, as in starvation, this balance is upset; glucose cannot provide adequate C_4 acids to oxidize the C_2 fragments from unsuppressed fatty acid oxidation, resulting in the accumulation and overflow of ketone bodies.

Regulation of Protein Metabolism

The high rate of protein turnover in animal cells makes regulation of protein synthesis a sensitive focal point for hormonal influence. The survival time for proteins may vary from the long-lived hemoglobins to the rapidly replenished inducible liver enzymes. There are four hormones with essentially anabolic effects; under appropriate dietary conditions they produce net protein synthesis and a positive nitrogen balance. Growth hormone is probably the most significant of these anabolic endocrines in the young animal. As shown in Figure 10.1, GH spares amino acids from degradative metabolism in many ways, reducing carbon utilization and lipogenesis, increasing amino acid transport, and finally increasing protein synthesis by stimulating the translational activity of the ribosomes. The action of insulin resembles that of GH, in that both can lead to a positive nitrogen balance and a stimulation of ribosomal activity. Insulin makes more carbohydrate available; thus, amino acids can be spared from gluconeogenesis and are more available for protein synthesis. The availability of intracellular amino acids in cells seems to be a highly relevant factor in controlling the rate of protein synthesis. Insulin also appears to have a more direct stimulatory effect on protein synthesis in the liver.

The thyroid hormones have an underlying effect on all metabolism. In thyroid deficiency, all metabolic interchanges proceed sluggishly. An excess of thyroid hormones leads to a general catabolic effect and a negative nitrogen balance. Carbohydrates and fats are inadequate for the excessive rate of metabolism; this leads to protein degradation and the misuse of carbon skeletons of amino acids. Normal levels of the thyroid hormone are required for adequate protein synthesis. This effect is probably mediated at the translational level in many (but not all) tissues.

The anabolic effects of testosterone are more specific, but affected areas include muscle, as well as those tissues in the male mammal involved in reproduction.

The hormones that are most significantly involved in protein degradation are the glucocorticoids, which can produce protein wasting and negative nigrogen balance. Amino acids are mobilized from most tissues and transported to the liver, where they are catabolized or used for protein formation. While the glucocorticoids stimulate protein synthesis in the liver, their catabolic effects on muscle and other tissues predominate. Excess thyroid hormones can promote catabolism by increasing the metabolic demand for all metabolites, thus resulting in a reduced supply of amino acids for protein synthesis.

10.2 MECHANISMS OF HORMONE ACTION

The mechanism of the action of the various hormones has challenged the imagination of biologists for over half a century and spurred numerous speculative suggestions. A distinction must be made at the outset between hormone induction and regulation of cell growth in the developing organism, and the hormonal control of adult cells. It would not be expected that identical or even similar mechanisms would govern both types of hormonal effects. In differentiation it appears that some of the genetic machinery of the cell must be involved. Over 30 years ago, in a Harvey Lecture, C. H. Danforth suggested the close interrelation of genes and hormones in biological processes. In 1960, Clever and Karlson reported a direct effect of ecdysone in causing puffing of the salivary gland chromosomes of the blowfly. Karlson and co-workers have related ecdysone effects to an RNA-dependent, induced synthesis of the enzyme DOPA decarboxylase. Evidence is accumulating that thyroid hormones and GH modify protein synthesis by affecting both the transcriptional and translational levels prior to the onset of amphibian metamorphosis and mammalian maturation. In hormone-induced differentiation, a permanent effect on the expressions of the genetic apparatus must result. For example, under the influence of the thyroid hormones, amphibian tadpoles are induced to make adult forms of hemoglobin, which completely replace tadpole hemoglobins. In typical hormonal control of differentiated systems, no genetic modification is involved.

In general, hormones comprise a regulatory device superimposed on the already existing controls of cellular metabolism. The absence of detailed knowledge concerning normal metabolic controls has delayed our understanding of the intimate details of hormone action. We can only integrate the various endocrine mechanisms in a general way, centering around a few basic ideas. However, all of these represent mechanisms that involve an amplification of the effect of a trace substance such as a hormone.

Most evidence supports the idea that hormones act directly on their target cells. One hypothesis, however—perhaps the simplest of those proposed to explain the action of hormones—suggests that hormones affect the rate at which metabolites and nutrients reach cells. This idea attempts to account for acute changes in substrate and water content of target tissues by the assumption that the demonstrated hyperemia that follows administration of some hormones (estrogen in the case of the uterus and LH in the case of the ovary) is due to the release of histamine; the release of this substance is held to be the primary action of the hormone. However, this hypothesis does not allow for the intense tissue specificity that is characteristic of hormonal response. Furthermore, recent work in several laboratories has shown that the dose of histamine needed to mimic the action of estrogen on the uterus is toxic to the various cells of the uterus, and that ovulation can occur in animals heavily dosed with antihistamine drugs.

Hormones and Membrane Transport

Over 40 years ago, Höber proposed that hormone action might affect membrane transport or cellular permeability. Changes in transport of ions, water, amino acids, and sugars have been observed for most of the hormones (Table 10.1). Frequently, a single hormone modifies the uptake of several metabolites; for example, insulin affects the transport of sugars, amino acids, and numerous inorganic ions. The permeability hypothesis is especially attractive since it can account for significantly altered behavior of cells without a major modification of the existent normal control mechanisms. For example, protein anabolism can be stimulated by higher amino acid availability. Rapidly growing cells and tissues have higher concentrations of free amino acids than do comparable cells growing more slowly. Tissues must obtain their essential amino acids exogenously, and the ability to synthesize the remaining amino acids is relatively limited. Thus, a hormone that increases the permeability of amino acids, and thus their availability to the cells, can also stimulate protein synthesis.

The need for intact cell membranes to demonstrate transport of materials into cells may explain the difficulty in finding suitable subcellular (homogenate) systems that can respond to hormones and account for their in vivo effects. Many hormone-

TABLE 10.1 SUMMARY OF MAJOR IN VIVO EFFECTS OF HORMONES ON TRANSPORT OF IMPORTANT METABOLITES[a]

Hormone	Metabolite, Tissue, and Effect[b]
ACTH	PO_4^{3-}, uric acid; renal transport (−) H_2O; mitochondria (+) Amino acids; adrenal (+), renal transport (+) Sugars; adrenal (+)
Aldosterone	Na^+; renal transport (+), toad bladder (+), frog skin (+) Blood cells (+), and other tissues (+)
Androgens	Na^+, K^+, others; renal transport (+) Amino acids; skeletal muscle (+), kidney (+), renal transport (+)
Calcitonin	Ca^{2+}; bone (+), kidney (−)
Epinephrine	Amino acids; heart (+), liver (+), kidney (+), intestine (+) Sugars; renal transport (+)
Estrogens	H_2O, Na^+, K^+; uterus (+) PO_4^{3-}; erythrocytes (−) I^-; thyroid (+) Amino acids; uterus (+), renal transport (−) Sugars; uterus (+), erythrocytes (−)
Glucagon	Sugars; adipose (+), diaphragm (+)
Glucocorticoids	Na^+; renal transport (+) PO_4^{3-}; renal transport (−) Ca^{2+}; intestinal absorption (−) Na^+; gill (+), nasal gland secretion (+) Amino acids; liver (+), diaphragm (−) Sugars; adipose (−), diaphragm (−)
Growth hormone	PO_4^{3-}, SO_4^{2-}; renal transport (+) H_2O: mitochrondria (+) Amino acids; skeletal muscle (+), heart (+), liver (+), diaphragm (+), adipose (+) Sugars; diaphragm (+), adipose (+)
Insulin	K^+, PO_4^{3-}; muscle, (in vitro) (+) Amino acids; most tissues (+), renal transport (−) Sugars; muscle (+) Na^+; muscle (in vitro) (−) H_2O; mitochondria (+)
Neurohypophyseal hormones	H_2O, Na^+ urea; renal tubule (+), toad bladder (+), skin (+) Sugars; adipose (+)
Parathormone	PO_4^{3-}; renal secretion (+), reabsorption (−) Ca^{2+} renal reabsorption (−), intestinal absorption (+)
Thyroid-stimulating hormone	I^- and others; thyroid (+) Amino acids; skin (+), muscle (+), liver (+), thyroid slices (+) Sugars; thyroid slices (+)
Thyroxin	H_2O; mitochondria (+)

[a]Table adapted from T. Riggs, G. Litwack and D. Kritchevsky (eds.), in *Mechanisms of Hormone Action*, Academic Press Inc., New York, 1964.
[b](+) = increase; (−) = decrease.

induced metabolic alterations have been impossible to reproduce in subcellular systems, perhaps due to destruction of the organization of the cell or its membranes. On the other hand, the effects of hormones may be explained by the increase in rate of transport.

Changes in amino acid transport initiated by glucocorticoids, insulin, and GH are clearly germane to the overall effect of these hormones. Variations in membrane permeability of essential ions have also been noted as effects of aldosterone, PTH, CT, and oxytocin administration.

Adenosine-cyclic-3',5'-monophosphate as the Second Messenger

The adenylcyclase system, which is a target for a number of hormones, is localized in the cell membrane (Figure 10.2); it is responsible for the formation of c-AMP from ATP. The hormone involved interacts in some unspecified way with

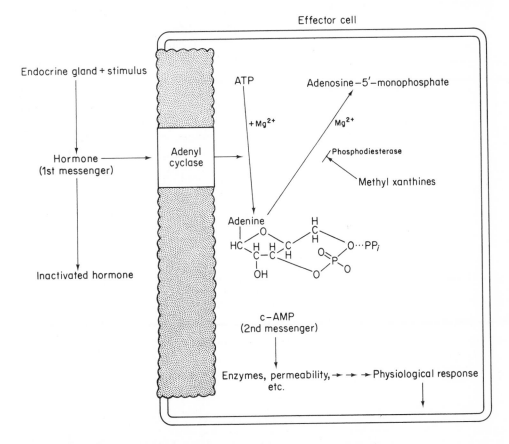

Figure 10.2 The second messenger system involving adenylcyclase. [Modified from E. W. Sutherland, G. Alan Robieson, and R. W. Butcher, "Some Aspects of the Biological Role of Adenosine 3',5'-Monophosphate (Cyclic AMP)," *Circulation*, 37, 279-306 (1968). By permission of the American Heart Association, Inc.]

the membrane of the affected cell to increase the activity of this system. Thus, the information provided by the extracellular signal of the first messenger, the hormone, is transmitted via a signal provided by the second messenger, c-AMP, which is capable of acting within the cell. The intracellular signal may be amplified in various ways, as dictated by the enzymic profile of the particular cell. Thus far, the only second messenger to be identified is c-AMP. It has been established as an intermediate in an impressive number of hormonal effects (Table 10.2). The generality of the role of c-AMP as a second signal leads to the suggestion that endocrine specificity must depend on the structure of the membrane receptor and the enzymic profile of the target tissues; c-AMP, the glucagon or epinephrine-induced metabolite, accounts for the glycogenolytic activities of these two hormones. The result of their action is magnified through a multiordered enzyme system consisting of the sequence of steps (see Figures 4.4 and 4.5) that begins with the increased activity of adenylcyclase resulting in the formation of c-AMP; this then causes a phosphorylation of phosphorylase b kinase, which in turn activates glycogen phosphorylase b to glycogen phosphorylase a. The net result is increased glycogenolysis and hyperglycemia. The catecholamines interact with membranes at specific receptor sites; two operationally defined sites have been described. It has also been suggested that the β receptors are part of the adenylcyclase system.

There is also the possibility of "anti"-second-messenger effects. The antilipolytic effect of insulin depends on its ability to inhibit the formation of c-AMP in adipose tissue. Prostaglandin,* a tissue "autacoid," first isolated from the prostate gland but now known to be present in many tissues, antagonizes c-AMP action in a variety of tissues. Prostaglandin is also known to block the lipolytic effects of epinephrine without affecting the metabolic or cardiovascular responses.

TABLE 10.2   SOME HORMONAL RESPONSES INVOLVING ADENOSINE-CYCLIC-3′,5′-MONOPHOSPHATE

Hormone	Response
Catecholamines	Phosphorylase activation (liver)
Epinephrines, etc.	Phosphorylase activation (heart)
	Positive inotropic response (heart)
	Lipolysis (adipose tissue)
Glucagon	Phosphorylase activation (liver)
	Insulin release (pancreas)
ACTH	Steroidogenesis (adrenal cortex)
LH (ICSH)	Steroidogenesis (corpus luteum)
Angiotensin	Steroidogenesis (zona glomerulosa)
Vasopressin	Permeability changes
TSH	Thyroid-hormone production
MSH	Melanocyte dispersion
Serotonin	Phosphofructokinase activation
Gastrin	HCl production

*Prostaglandin, first isolated from the prostate gland, has now been shown to be ubiquitously distributed in many tissues.

Enzymes and Hormones

Besides the cell membrane a limited number of sites are available for the action of hormones, but in all situations an amplifying mechanism must be involved. The classical source of intracellular amplification is the enzymes. When the full significance of the action of enzymes, vitamins, and minerals as coenzymes was first appreciated several decades ago, it was optimistically hoped that the last remaining group of unexplained trace-substance effects—those due to hormone action—could be interpreted in terms of the well-known components of cellular enzymic machinery. However, it is still not possible to account for hormone action in terms of interaction with a specific enzyme or enzymes. Perhaps it was too much to expect that the specificity and multiplicity of hormone action could be explained by such an oversimplified mechanism. The most popular example of an inferred enzymic effect is the previously cited glucagon and epinephrine stimulation of adenylcyclase, which increases the intracellular level of c-AMP. The molecular details of these reactions, however, have remained elusive because of both the difficulty in isolating and purifying a key enzyme, adenylcyclase, and the possible involvement of the cell membrane in the activating mechanism.

An impressive number of in vitro effects of hormones on enzyme systems have filled the endocrinological and biochemical literature. These data suffer from two major criticisms.

(1) The concentrations of hormones needed are frequently much greater than are the in vivo concentrations. For example, the purported in vitro effects of T_3 on c-AMP systems in adipose tissue were achieved at concentrations of 10^{-3} to 10^{-4} M, fully 10^3 to 10^5 times greater than the estimated normal overall tissue concentrations of 10^{-7} to 10^{-8} M. A molecule such as T_3 or T_4, with a variety of functional groups (such as phenolic OH and I), might be expected to affect many systems nonspecifically at concentrations of 10^{-3} to 10^{-4} M.

(2) The in vitro enzymic effects have not been successfully related to the recognized in vivo effects of the hormones. The interesting reactions (shown below) studied by Talalay, Villee, Williams-Ashman, and their co-workers, of 17β-hydroxysteroid (estradiol) dehydrogenases yielding NADH and NADP$^+$, in which the steroid hormone serves as a transhydrogenase coenzyme, have not proved relevant to estrogen action.

$$\text{estradiol} + \text{NAD}^+ \rightleftharpoons \text{estrone} + \text{NADH} + \text{H}^+$$
$$\text{estrone} + \text{NADPH} + \text{H}^+ \rightleftharpoons \text{estradiol} + \text{NADP}^+$$

net reaction:
$$\text{NADPH} + \text{NAD}^+ \rightleftharpoons \text{NADP}^+ + \text{NADH}$$

A possible mechanism for hormonal control by interaction with enzymes has emerged from the proposals by Monod *et al.* concerning allosteric effectors. This theory suggests that the interaction of low-molecular-weight effector substances with proteins leads to changes in their function and physical state, even though the effector substance is not involved in the functioning of the protein. These proteins, which Monod has called "allosteric" proteins, include those which take part in certain systems involved in the control of genetic expression, protein synthesis, and enzyme induction. For example, the allosteric protein might react with the genetic material of the chromosomes, repressing its ability to serve as a template for RNA synthesis. A low-molecular-weight effector such as a hormone might then modify this allosteric protein's ability to repress RNA synthesis, thereby causing induction. Despite the attractiveness of this hypothesis and the demonstration that many hormones can interact with a variety of proteins, no authentic application of the hypothesis has yet been found.

Hormones and Protein Biosynthesis

The theory that hormones may act directly upon the transcription and translation processes involved in protein biosynthesis has received considerable experimental support. The flow of information that determines the kind of proteins synthesized is known to involve the three basic processes depicted in Figure 10.3: replication, transcription, and translation.

The replication process, in which deoxyribonucleotides are assembled linearly to form identical sequences of the original chromosomal DNA, usually can be involved when permanent differentiation occurs, as in metamorphosis and sexual develop-

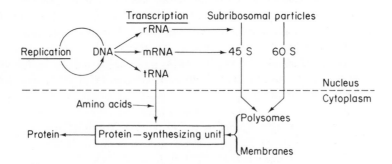

Figure 10.3 A simplified scheme showing the biosynthetic relationships between the nucleic acids (DNA and RNA) and proteins that determine information flow and protein synthesis in nucleated cells. As discussed in more detail in the text, the transcription and translation processes are the logical sites of hormone action. It has been further proposed that the type of growth or development would be determined genetically via mRNA coding for specific proteins but that its expression requires the generation of ribosomes and their topographical segregation by firm attachment to membranes. [Modified from J. R. Tata, "Hormonal Regulation of Growth and Protein Synthesis," *Nature,* **219**, 331-337 (1968).]

ment. But in the typical hormone-dominated process there is no modification of the kind of cell produced after hormone treatment.

In transcription, a specific DNA sequence is transcribed into the complementary RNA sequence. Although all RNA's are functional constituents of the final translation mechanism, it is the messenger, mRNA, that carries the information specifying the amino acid sequence of the protein product. Thus, either modified or new mRNA might produce a new and unique protein or proteins.

One of the earliest proposals, made by P. Karlson in 1963 (Figure 10.4), was based on the Jacob and Monod model for enzyme induction in bacteria. It was suggested that hormones activate genes by acting as inducers, which by combining with appropriate repressors, control mRNA synthesis and thus regulate protein synthesis. The hormone molecules may not work directly on the repressor-chromosome complex. Recent work suggests that hormones bind to specific protein molecules in responsive cells. It is believed this hormone-protein complex interacts with the chromosome, causing the derepression of specific and appropriate parts of the genome.

Growth hormone, estrogens, testosterone, glucocorticoids, and the thyroid hormones all show an effect on some aspect of RNA biosynthesis in responsive tissues. But it has yet to be convincingly demonstrated that this RNA increase is specifically related to an identifiable mRNA. The most relevant experimental claims include: (1) alteration of enzyme activity of adrenals and ovaries maintained in organ culture by RNA extracted from either the adrenal or testis of rats (the pattern of steroid hormone synthesis of the cultured endocrine tissue reflects the origin of the RNA); (2) induction of uterine growth by the intrauterine addition of RNA from estrogen-activated tissue; (3) induction of tyrosine-α-ketoglutarate transaminase activity in an in vitro protein-synthesizing system from rat liver by a liver RNA fraction from cortisol-treated rats; and (4) induction of DOPA decarboxylase activity in the blowfly by RNA preparations from ecdysone-treated insects. As described later, a more complex mechanism has been devised to account for the role of RNA at the translational level.

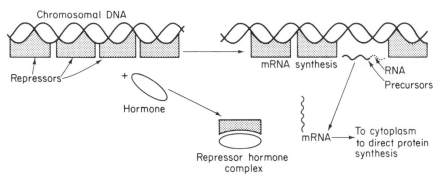

Figure 10.4 Induction of the synthesis of a new protein by a hormone acting as a derepressor. [Modified from P. Karlson, "New Concepts in the Mode of Action of Hormones," *Perspectives Biol. Med.*, 6, 203 (1963). Copyright © 1963 by the University of Chicago Press.]

Translational control provides another mechanism that may operate independently of hormone-induced changes in the rate of RNA biosynthesis. In the translational process, the coded information, coming originally from DNA and contained in mRNA, programs the ribosomes for synthesis of specific protein molecules. The steps from mRNA to protein are a complex series of reactions, all involved in the translation of the four-unit nucleotide language of RNA into the twenty-unit amino acid language of amino acid sequences of protein.

The synthesis of other macromolecules (fats, carbohydrates, and so forth) is directly dependent on protein enzymes with specific structures and thus more indirectly related to the cell's hereditary material, DNA. Therefore, if hormones were to increase the translational activity of certain ribosomes, the protein profile of a cell could be shifted in the direction(s) dictated by particular hormones. Combinations of these various effects could produce the multiplicity of hormone actions so frequently encountered.

As often happens, particularly in the higher animal, a more complex mechanism of hormone action is emerging. It has become increasingly clear that the Jacob-Monod proposals to describe microbial genetics and enzyme inductions must be modified when applied to vertebrate enzyme systems. It is now believed that mRNA in nucleated cells is transported from the nucleus to the cytoplasm while complexed with ribosomes. The mRNA-ribosomal complex is integrated with a larger ribosomal component to form a polysome. Several major effects of action within the translational machinery have been proposed by Tata and co-workers for hormones involved in growth and development (Figure 10.3). These include: (1) stimulation of synthesis of ribosomal and nuclear RNA; (2) acceleration of the rate of formation of ribosomal precursor particles; (3) increase in the transport to the cytoplasm of the ribosome subunits with attached mRNA; (4) buildup of new polyribosomes in the cytoplasm with different protein products; and (5) perhaps the regulation of the possible role of the cell membrane in correctly orienting mRNA in relation to the ribosomes to which it is bound. Table 10.3 summarizes examples of marked stimulation of RNA biosynthesis in the nucleus by several hormones. In the absence of specific data supporting mRNA biosynthesis, a more general type of nuclear RNA effect could be interpreted as an increase in ribosomal turnover. Similarly, the increase in RNA polymerase activity has been associated with an RNA product that resembles the ribosomal type more closely. This has led Tata, Hamilton, and others to propose that one or more steps in the translational function of the ribosomes might be sensitive to endocrines.

10.3 FINAL SUMMARY

Any metazoan cell floating in a sea of intercellular fluid can perform a myriad of chemical processes as long as its environment can be maintained in a compatible equilibrium. Hormones increase the availability and utilization of organic and inorganic metabolites by cells that, acting together as organs, can regulate the

TABLE 10.3   STIMULATION OF RNA BIOSYNTHESIS IN VARIOUS TISSUES
AFTER TREATMENT WITH HORMONES[a]

Hormone	Animal	Tissue	System Stimulated
Growth hormone	Hypophysectomized rat	Liver	Rapidly labeled RNA in vivo; RNA polymerase
	Hypophysectomized, castrated rat	Muscle	RNA polymerase
Thyroid hormones	Thyroidectomized rat	Liver	Rapidly labeled RNA in vivo; RNA polymerase
	Bullfrog tadpole	Liver	RNA in vivo
Testosterone	Castrated rat	Prostate	Rapidly labeled RNA in vivo; RNA polymerase
	Hypophysectomized, castrated rat	Muscle	RNA polymerase
	Castrated rat	Liver	RNA polymerase
Estradiol	Ovariectomized rat	Uterus	Rapidly labeled RNA; RNA polymerase
Cortisone	Rat	Liver	45S ribosomal precursor

[a]Modified from J. R. Tata, *Biochem. J.,* **104** 4 (1967).

composition of the internal environment. Hormones may affect the transport of solutes across membranes and the metabolism of those metabolites, which are principal sources of energy. They may initiate these effects directly, in a presently poorly understood manner, or indirectly, by generating a second messenger or modifying genetic expression, particularly in the translational and transcriptional phases of protein synthesis. Currently we have only a qualitative understanding of the biological machinery that achieves this regulation. A major objective of biochemical research of the future will be to elaborate and quantitate the cellular mechanisms by which the hormones exert their effects.

REFERENCES

Hechter, O., and I. D. K. Halkerston: "On the Action of Mammalian Hormones," in G. Pincus and K. V. Thimann (eds.), *The Hormones,* vol. 5, pp. 697-825, Academic Press, Inc., New York, 1964.

Karlson, P., and C. E. Sekeris: "Biochemical Mechanisms of Hormone Action," *Acta Endocrinol.,* **53**, 505-518 (1966).

Litwack, G. (ed.): *Biochemical Actions of Hormones,* Academic Press, Inc., New York, 1970.

Tata, J. R.: "Hormonal Regulation of Growth and Protein Synthesis," *Nature,* **219**, 331 (1968).

APPENDIX COMMONLY OCCURRING AMINO ACIDS AND THEIR ABBREVIATIONS

Amino Acids	Abbreviations
1. Aliphatic amino acids	
Glycine	gly
Alanine	ala
Valine	val
Leucine	leu
Isoleucine	ile
2. Hydroxyamino acids	
Serine	ser
Threonine	thr
3. Dicarboxylic amino acids and their amides	
Aspartic acid	asp
Asparagine	$aspNH_2$ or asn
Glutamic acid	glu
Glutamine	$gluNH_2$ or gln
4. Amino acids having basic functions	
Lysine	lys
Hydroxylysine	hylys
Histidine	his
Arginine	arg
5. Aromatic amino acids (histidine included in category 4)	
Phenylalanine	phe
Tyrosine	tyr
Tryptophan	try
Thyroxine	T_4
6. Sulfur-containing amino acids	
Cysteine	cySH
Cystine	cyS–Syc
Methionine	met
7. Imino acids	
Proline	pro
Hydroxyproline	hypro

INDEX